The Complete Guide to

MEDICAID AND NURSING HOME COSTS

How to Keep Your Family Assets Protected

Up to Date Medicaid Secrets You Need to Know

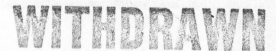

The Complete Guide to Medicaid and Nursing Home Costs: How to Keep Your Family Assets Protected: Up to Date Medicaid Secrets You Need to Know

Copyright © 2008 by Atlantic Publishing Group, Inc.
1405 SW 6th Ave. • Ocala, Florida 34471 • 800-814-1132 • 352-622-1875–Fax
Web site: www.atlantic-pub.com • E-mail: sales@atlantic-pub.com
SAN Number: 268-1250

ISBN-13: 978-1-60138-153-8   ISBN-10: 1-60138-153-0

Library of Congress Cataloging-in-Publication Data

The complete guide to Medicaid and nursing home costs : how to keep your family assets protected : up to date Medicaid secrets you need to know.
    p. cm.
Includes bibliographical references and index.
ISBN-13: 978-1-60138-153-8 (alk. paper)
ISBN-10: 1-60138-153-0 (alk. paper)
1. Medicaid. 2. Nursing homes--Rates--United States.

RA412.4.C66 2008
368.4'200973--dc22
            2008016050

INTERIOR LAYOUT DESIGN: Nicole Deck • ndeck@atlantic-pub.com

Printed in the United States

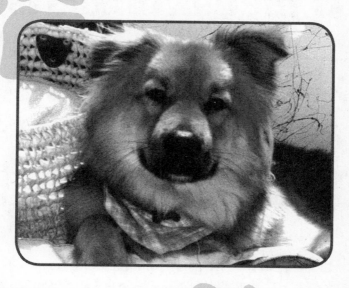

We recently lost our beloved pet, Bear, who was not only our best and dearest friend, but also the "Vice President of Sunshine" here at Atlantic Publishing. He did not receive a salary, but worked tirelessly 24 hours a day to please his parents. Bear was a rescue dog who turned around and showered myself, my wife Sherri, his grandparents Jean, Bob, and Nancy and every person and animal he met (maybe not rabbits) with friendship and love. He made a lot of people smile every day.

We wanted you to know that a portion of the profits of this book will be donated to the Humane Society of the United States.

–Douglas & Sherri Brown

THE HUMANE SOCIETY
OF THE UNITED STATES ©

The human-animal bond is as old as human history. We cherish our animal companions for their unconditional affection and acceptance. We feel a thrill when we glimpse wild creatures in their natural habitat or in our own backyard.

Unfortunately, the human-animal bond has at times been weakened. Humans have exploited some animal species to the point of extinction.

The Humane Society of the United States makes a difference in the lives of animals here at home and worldwide. The HSUS is dedicated to creating a world where our relationship with animals is guided by compassion. We seek a truly humane society in which animals are respected for their intrinsic value, and where the human-animal bond is strong.

Want to help animals? We have plenty of suggestions. Adopt a pet from a local shelter, join The Humane Society and be a part of our work to help companion animals and wildlife. You will be funding our educational, legislative, investigative and outreach projects in the U.S. and across the globe.

Or perhaps you'd like to make a memorial donation in honor of a pet, friend or relative? You can through our Kindred Spirits program. And if you'd like to contribute in a more structured way, our Planned Giving Office has suggestions about estate planning, annuities, and even gifts of stock that avoid capital gains taxes.

Maybe you have land that you would like to preserve as a lasting habitat for wildlife. Our Wildlife Land Trust can help you. Perhaps the land you want to share is a backyard—that's enough. Our Urban Wildlife Sanctuary Program will show you how to create a habitat for your wild neighbors.

So you see, it's easy to help animals. And The HSUS is here to help.

The Humane Society of the United States
2100 L Street NW
Washington, DC 20037
202-452-1100
www.hsus.org

Table of Contents

Chapter 1: Medicaid   15

What Is Medicaid? 15

Home- and Community-Based Living Programs
Under Medicaid 19

Medicaid Care Coordination..............................23

Chapter 2: Resources of the Single or Married Applicant   33

Determining Value of Assets 33

What Are the 50 and 100 Percent States? 39

The Snapshot Rule 40

Split Transfers 40

Chapter 3: Medicaid Estate Recovery   43

A Brief History of Estate Recovery 43

Estate Recovery Trends in Individual States................50

Chapter 4: Asset Protection Strategies for Those Applying to Medicaid   55

Transferring Assets: Tips for Doing It the Right Way 55

Trusts and Medicaid 56

Revocable and Irrevocable Trusts: What They Are
and What They Do 63

Self-Settled and Pooled Trusts 65

Irrevocable Life Insurance Trust Pros and Cons 66

Charitable Remainder Trusts 69

529 Plans and Medicaid: How They Work 70

Advanced Directives 72

Chapter 5: Annuities   79

What Are Annuities? 79

Medicaid Annuities 80

Annuities and Medicaid 81

Types of Annuities 83

Tips for Single Persons Purchasing Annuities for
Medicaid 86

Tips for Married Couples Purchasing Medicaid
Annuities 88

Chapter 6: Gifts   91

Medicaid Penalty Periods 92

Value of the Gift 93

Look-Back Period 94

Gift Splitting 96

Gift Trusts 97

Long-Term Life Insurance and Gifts 97

Gift Taxes 100

Cons of Long-Term Health Insurance 101

Generation-Skipping Transfer Tax 101

Chapter 7: Wills and Deeds   103

What Should Be in a Will? 104

Different Types of Wills 105

Changing or Challenging a Will 106

Lady Bird Deeds or Enhanced Life Estate Deeds....107

Beneficiary Deeds 109

Joint Owners with Rights of Survivorship 110

Executors and Trustees 111

Chapter 8: Creative Ways to Qualify for Medicaid   115

Tips on Medicaid Spend Down...............................117

Long-Term Care Insurance 120

Irrevocable Life Insurance 122

Spousal Refusal 124

Children as Paid Caregivers 125

Warnings on Limited Family Partnerships 129

Chapter 9: What to Do With Your Home 133

Keep It, Sell It or Transfer House to Kids? 134

Life Estates 139

Purchase a Joint Interest in a Child's Home 140

Child Moves into Your Home 141

Parent Moves into the Home 143

Taxes on the Home..146

Chapter 10: Where to Contact Your State Agency   147

Medicaid News from State to State 166

Chapter 11: How to Transfer Gifts   225

Old Half-a-Loaf Method 225

New Half-a-Loaf Methods...225

Exceptions to the Rule for Transferring Gifts..................226

Trust for Sole Benefit of Spouse, Blind or Disabled Child, or Person Under Age 65 227

Transfers for Non-Medicaid Reasons...............................228

Chapter 12: Promissory Notes Explained   231

Interest Rate Charged on Notes.......................................233

New Rules on Promissory Notes.......................................233

Chapter 13: Alternative Services to Nursing Homes   **237**

Home Care Programs 237

Assisted Living Centers 241

Adult Daycare...247

Adult Day Healthcare Options 251

Taking Care of Your Parents or Elderly Relatives in Your Home or Theirs 255

Alternative Healthcare 263

Chapter 14: How to Find a Good Elder Lawyer   **265**

What Is Elder Law?...265

What Is Certification and Is It Important?.......................266

Tips for Preparing to Meet an Elder Lawyer.................267

Chapter 15: Alzheimer's Disease and Medicaid   **269**

Financial Planning with Alzheimer's Disease 270

Types of Long-term Care for Alzheimer's Patients........272

Case Studies   **275**

Bibliography   **281**

Index   **283**

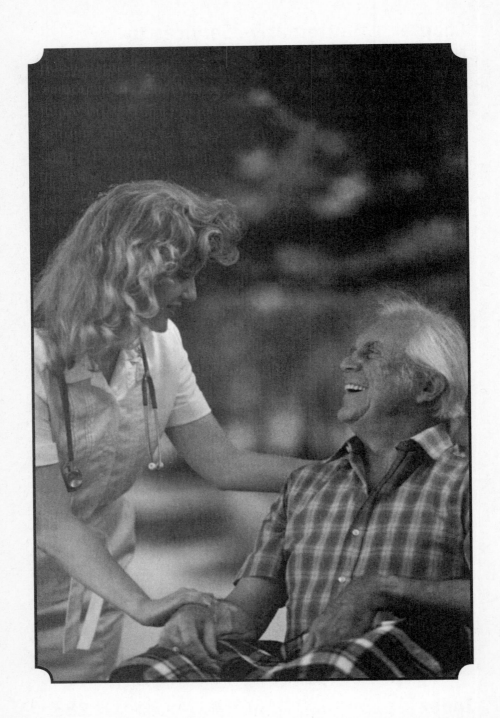

Introduction

The monthly cost of nursing home care is rising each year, ranging from $6,757.67 in Pennsylvania to $9,096 in Connecticut for 2008. Medicare does not cover long-term nursing home costs; neither does most healthcare insurance. So if you develop a long-term chronic illness that requires medical insurance, the only program that might pay your expenses is Medicaid. That is, if you qualify with the strict low-income requirements that most states have.

The cost of long-term medical care can wipe out your family savings and assets, costing you thousands of dollars. This book is about Medicaid and learning how to plan so you can protect your assets and home. You will learn the latest laws and techniques to help you plan. Consult an elder-care lawyer when planning for long-term health problems. Elder-care lawyers can help you plan how to save your assets and eventually qualify for Medicaid. They know the new rules and regulations and the latest techniques available.

There are many different laws, and Medicaid can be extremely confusing. Each state handles Medicaid differently, so it is important to plan and get professional help. This book will help you understand the issues, and prepare you to consult with an elder-care lawyer or deal with the Medicaid agency yourself. The book will tell you about other long-term care programs and services available to the elderly. This varies from state to state, but you will get a good overview of the range of services available.

Take the time to plan wisely for your senior years. Consult an elder-care lawyer to help you with Medicaid planning. New laws allowing the state to put a lien on your home if you or a family member qualifies for Medicaid make it harder to hold on to your money. The state also can file a claim after a Medicaid recipient dies — another reason to consult an expert.

This book will give you the information you need so when you decide to consult with an elder-care attorney, you will know enough about the subject to make some wise decisions. You will know if the lawyer you consult truly knows the subject. Consult someone active in the field who knows the changing laws; someone who works with families and older clients and has real experience.

Medicaid is now offering some home-based programs for the elderly that allow them to live at home. This is offered in some states as an alternative to long-term care. Improving health and wellness will become a focus as the years go on, so you can save money from the financial debt of the nursing homes. Many programs are being monitored for cost-effectiveness, so this will change some of the rules for Medicaid assets and eligibility. For a full list of eligibility requirements visit **http:// www.cms.hhs.gov/MedicaidEligibility/09_SpousalImpov- erishment.asp.**

Introduction

The Home and Community Based Services (HCBS) programs are offered under the Medicaid waiver program for elderly and disabled persons as alternatives to going into long-term care. It is a viable option that may become a better alternative than the nursing home.

There is now a five-year look-back period for the transferring of assets. A person cannot apply for Medicaid until five years from the date of transferring assets. It used be three years, and this period may become even longer. Still, you can learn about the laws and make the best choices by consulting an elder-care lawyer who knows how to prepare and advise you on these complicated issues.

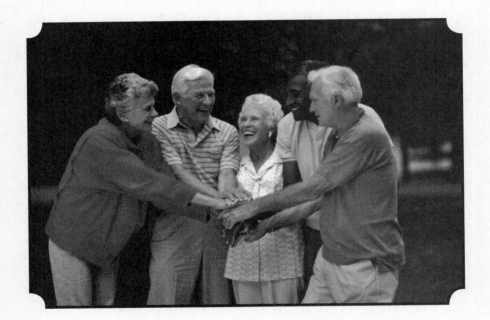

CHAPTER 1

Medicaid

What Is Medicaid?

Medicaid is a program run by the federal government and individual states that provides medical coverage to low-income or poor individuals and families. These people commonly have no insurance or inadequate insurance to cover their needs. Each state has its own Medicaid office, so the different states have different laws that determine who qualifies. The program has different names in some states, such as Medical Assistance or Med-Cal.

Low-income women, children, and elderly are some of the groups that fit into the Medicaid program. Blind, disabled, caretakers, low-income pregnant women, and elderly persons who need long-term care such as nursing homes often qualify for this program. Anyone who qualifies for Medicaid must meet certain strict requirements.

Medicaid was established in 1965, about the same time as Medicare, as part of the Social Security Act Amendments. This amendment established Medicare, a health insurance program for the elderly and Medicaid, a health insurance program for the poor. The federal government funds most of Medicaid and often gives more money to poorer states. Average elderly individuals and couples do not qualify for this program. They have a home, reasonable income, and other assets. Yet, Medicaid is one of the only programs that covers nursing homes costs. If you were to become ill and had to go to a nursing home, the cost could wipe out your savings and assets. The average monthly cost of a nursing home per month for one person ranges from $6757.67 to $9096.

There is a joint program for Medicaid and Medicare called Program of All-Inclusive Care for the Elderly (PACE). It may be available in some states that choose it as an optional Medicaid benefit. PACE is an option instead of care through a nursing home. To qualify, you must be 55 or older, live in the service area, and be certified by the state as eligible for nursing home care. Check with your Medicaid agency to see if there is a PACE program near you.

How Medicaid Works with Medicare

Medicaid pays Medicare Part B premiums and deductibles if an eligible person does not have secondary insurance. It is a supplemental insurance for the elderly already on Medicare who need further assistance due to low income. It also covers extended nursing home care.

Medicare is a federally funded program, providing medical coverage for people 65 and older. It covers elderly who are disabled. Medicare Part A covers inpatient services such as hospital care and 100 days of care in a nursing home. It also covers care for terminally ill patients.

Medicare pays only limited nursing home care for patients who require a limited stay to recuperate from an illness; it does not provide for long-term nursing care. Medicare Part B is optional and individuals pay for the plan through deductions from their Social Security checks. It covers preventive care, tests, screening, physicians' services, and other basic medical services.

Medicaid is not available to everyone 65 or older. It is based on strict income guidelines and need. It works with Medicaid to fill in gaps not covered by Medicare.

The PACE program is modeled after long-term care and acute services developed by Lok Senior Healthcare Services of California. The program was tested in the 1980s and was developed to address needs of long-term care clients, providers, and programs that paid for the services. For many participants, it allows them to remain at home instead of being put in nursing home or long-term care facility.

The Balanced Budget Act established the PACE program as a permanent part of Medicare and allows states to provide PACE services to Medicaid applicants. The state plan must include PACE as an optional Medicaid benefit before the individual state can participate in programs with PACE providers.

Participants in the PACE program must be 55 years or older, live in the state, and be certified for nursing home care by the state agency. This program became the sole program for Medicare and Medicaid eligible enrollees. A team assesses the needs of individual participants for services. It provides primarily social and medical services for adult daycare centers, and in-home services. The providers receive Medicare and Medicaid monthly payments if they qualify. The average time it takes to process a PACE application is nine months. Some of the services covered are prescriptions drugs, hospice care, and mental-health services.

Individuals who are covered by Medicare Part A or B and by part of Medicaid are known as dual eligibles. People who have Medicare and limited income may get help from Medicaid for paying out-of-pocket medical expenses or what Medicare does not cover. This dual program is sometimes called the Medicare Savings Program. Services that are covered by Medicare will first be paid by this program, and the balance is paid by Medicaid.

What Is Covered Under Medicaid

Medicaid will pay most medical bills once a person has been approved. People who are covered by Medicare and Medicaid, known as dual eligibles, are covered for nursing home stays, prescription drugs, hospital visits, and more. Medical coverage varies from state to state, but most coverage includes inpatient and outpatient hospital services, doctor services, medical and surgical dental services, lab and X-ray, nursing facility services for those 21 or older, and family nurse practitioner services.

Some services are optional, but most states under Medicaid will offer ambulance service to those in nursing homes, prescription drug coverage, eye doctor visits, glasses, prosthetic devices, dental, and in-home assistance.

If you qualify and are living at home, Medicaid will pay for some services. Some states have the HCBS program. Most states now can offer this program without applying for a waiver through the federal government. Check with your state to see if it offers this plan and what it will cover. Program coverage includes homemaker and home health aides, personal-care services, adult day health services, rehabilitation for safety, hygiene, housekeeping, and case management.

HCBS may apply to certain services at assisted living centers. Assisted living centers must be Medicaid certified to be covered. HCBS will not cover basic room and board because assisted living centers are not considered nursing homes.

When a person is qualified, Medicaid will pay the full cost of nursing home bills. This includes room, meals, and all medical services. Some nursing homes do not accept Medicaid payment. If you or a family member move into a nursing home, find out if Medicaid is accepted. Nursing homes that do not accept Medicaid payment require the patient to transfer to another facility if money or private-pay options run out. It can be awfully upsetting for a patient to have to move suddenly after getting comfortable at a nursing home.

Home- and Community-Based Living Programs Under Medicaid

Changes are underway to reform Medicaid programs for the elderly. Many states are offering home- and community-based services as an option for Medicaid recipients. This means they will not be in a nursing home, but will get help that assists them in continuing to live at home alone or with a family member. There is a trend of some states offering options or programs other than nursing home care because it is so expensive.

New Jersey passed an act in 2005 to find a better balance between long-term care and community-based services. The state is looking for models that are cost-effective alternatives to living in a nursing home.

Vermont has developed a program where spouses may now be paid to care for family members. There is an option for 24-hour in-home care using a home provider or shared living arrangement. Vermont has monitored the program and continues to look for other community-based programs that are cost-effective. In Idaho, a reform initiative seeks to encourage preventive treatment and provide alternative treatment to the elderly. It includes case management, dental, vision, transportation, and extensive mental-health services for individuals with developmental disabilities.

The state of Alabama departments of Medicaid, senior services, and rehab services have a program that provides a money allowance for which individuals can determine what services they need. Elderly people can choose who to hire for their care and save money for equipment purchases. Consumers decide who provides care and when it is needed. They develop and follow a spending plan, and hire and manage their support staff.

This shift from long-term care to community-based care is the trend. HCBS waivers give states funds for services that do not fit the typical Medicaid long-term programs. Some of the services are case management, homemakers, personal-attendant care, home health aide services, adult daycare services, transportation, home-delivered meals, and respite care.

Texas plans to assist individuals who go from nursing homes to community-based programs. This may include some elderly who have behavioral health conditions. For those in nursing homes, the state will build on services that are home and community based. The state of Washington wants to assist older adults who want to move from an institution to their own communities.

A program called Money Follows the Person gives the secretary of U. S. Health and Human Services the right to award competitive grants to increase the use of HCBS services. It supports people who want to move from the nursing home, or other facility, back into community. Some states have targeted the aging population.

HCBS services include adult daycare, providing services five days a week during normal business hours, and also meals and social interaction for seniors and other disabled persons. Some HCBS plans have nurses or social workers — case managers designed to assist the family or member. They develop long-term care plans and monitor them.

HCBS services are regulated under a Medicaid waiver that allows individual states to pick a wide range of home and community services for the elderly. This program began in 1981 under section 1915(c) of the Social Security Act. HCBS provides these services by waiving certain Medicaid statutes and regulations. It is designed to enable elderly who are at risk to be placed in long-term care to remain in their homes. This preserves the elderly person's sense of independence and control over his or her environment. Most states now have some form of this program under Medicaid.

Nutritional services are included under this program, such as home-delivered meals, nutritional counseling, dietetic instruction, and nutritional assessment. The nutritional services help reduce risk in the elderly population using case management.

Providers for these programs must meet certain criteria. They must be licensed assisted living centers, home health agencies, meal delivery services, local health departments, and other such agencies. Nutritional services must be licensed nutritionists, dieticians, home health agencies, hospitals, and services approved to participate in Medicaid.

This Medicaid waiver program provides choices for individuals to pick their own provider for the medical services they are eligible for. This gives elderly people living at home again more control over their lives, which means a better lifestyle for everyone. Choices may be limited depending on the program the state offers. The services from this program serve the elderly who are fragile and need more services, but do not qualify for a nursing home.

Respite services are available for short periods to give regular caregivers some relief. Many HCBS recipients live with their adult children or alone, and need help to do daily tasks. The Medicaid Adult Daycare program provides services to adults age 16 and older, including the elderly. It is a structured program that provides health, social, and related support services. It allows those who live in the community to receive care during the day in a social group environment, and gives respite to caregivers at home.

More states are incorporating these services to keep the elderly out of nursing homes, and to help them remain independent and living at home.

Medicaid Care Coordination

Medicaid Care Coordination is a service that assesses the needs of a client and coordinating services that are appropriate to meet that client's needs. Some states use this service with Medicaid to improve the quality of care. The strongest trend is to have care coordination to improve and streamline care for individual clients. Arizona has a program for elderly who are at risk of having to go into a nursing home. The members can move between the two programs as needed. California provides a program for those who are seriously ill. The state strives to improve health and decrease long-term costs of the chronically ill by using a holistic approach. California provides disease management, financial and social support, and referrals to improve mobility. Kentucky uses the services of the private sector, universities, providers, and others, to support the overall care coordination and utilization of supplies and services. The program offers medical services in areas of diabetes, asthma, adult obesity, and heart initiatives.

Some programs provide personal assistance, adult foster care, adaptive aids, medical supplies, respite care, emergency response, and therapies.

Here are some examples of successful case management programs in Minnesota:

- A case manager was helping an elderly woman living at home. The elderly woman had mental problems and a severe skin condition that was worsening. She refused to go to her doctor because she feared leaving the neighborhood and the doctor was out of the region. The case manager arranged for her to see a doctor in the area. She went to the specialist and her skin condition improved, allowing her to live at home independently.

- A fragile 88-year-old woman was living at home with the help of services and family. She needed several items to remain at home, such as a raised toilet seat, wheelchair, grab bars in the shower, a walker, and bath transfer bench. The care coordinator was able to get her supplies, helping family caregivers take care of the woman at home. Her care coordinator bought her a blender, as she needed puréed food and better nutrition.

- A 74-year-old man had diabetes and heart disease. He had trouble keeping himself and his home clean and eating right. He was hospitalized several times before he was enrolled in the managed care program. His coordinator arranged meals on wheels, a home health aide, housekeeping, and skilled nursing. His health and outlook improved, and he has not been hospitalized since he began the program.

- Mrs. J. has a history of heart problems and being tired all the time. After Mrs. J. underwent triple bypass surgery, the coordinator arranged a temporary nursing home stay for her. Her family was unable to provide her with the care she needed. The coordinator did all the paperwork and worked with a nursing home to make sure Mrs. J. was recovering. When Mrs. J. returned home, the coordinator arranged housekeeping services and registered nurse services visits.

When and Where to Apply

You apply for benefits at the agency in your state that manages Medicaid. It varies from state to state, but all states have an agency that administers the program. You can write, call, or go in person to your state department of human services or social services. People on supplemental security income or old-age pension automatically receive Medicaid.

You can find contact information for these agencies in the government-issued blue book or your local phone book. Chapter 10 in this book has a list of Medicaid agencies by state. Some of the agencies are called by different names, such as the Department of Health and Social Services; Healthcare Cost Containment; Department of Health Services; Healthcare Policy and Financing; Human Services Division; Agency Healthcare Administration; Department of Community Health; Family and Social Service Administration; Department of Health and Hospital; and the Department of Health and Mental Hygiene.

When you apply too early, you often are ruled ineligible for Medicaid benefits. You may have to spend your assets or money before you qualify. This can cost you and your family thousands of dollars in medical bills. It is important to apply only when you think you or a family member will need Medicaid. Often, it is wise to consult an elder-law attorney who can help you qualify without losing all your assets. Another mistake some older people make is giving away their money or home too early. Sometimes, this causes tax problems and Medicaid complications that affect eligibility. Gifts can, at times, cause periods of ineligibility for Medicaid benefits.

When someone applies too late, that person may lose the opportunity to have nursing home costs and medical bills paid. This can result in the loss of your assets, home, savings, and other investments. Many individuals have lost all their money to a nursing home and state after becoming chronically ill. Poor planning can mean many months of not being eligible.

When applying for Medicaid, you have to provide income and asset information. You need records of bank accounts, insurance, investments, deeds, and trusts. To avoid delays, collect the necessary information before you apply. You may need information going back five years, so income tax returns are good documents to retain.

When applying for Medicaid, secure documentation proving you are a U.S. citizen. Acceptable documents are a U.S. passport, valid state driver's license, birth certificate, school ID card with photo, military card, or draft record. These documents should be originals or copies certified by the issuing agency.

If you or a relative apply for Medicaid at a nursing home, the nursing home may not expect you to pay until you find out if you qualify. Avoid paying the nursing home during the application process because it is hard to get a refund. You can appeal a rejection of Medicaid, especially if the person is in a nursing home to stay.

An applicant must meet medical qualifications to qualify for Medicaid. A person must prove to be at least 65 years old, blind, or disabled. Disabled is defined as not being able to do any gainful physical or mental activity that is caused by physical or mental impairment. Disability can result in death or is expected to last more than 12 months. Often, a trained nurse or worker will come to an applicant's home to determine if they are indeed disabled. The applicant must fail a certain number of tests to be determined qualified. Applicants can be turned down due to too many assets.

Medicaid Financial Qualifications

To qualify for Medicaid, a single person must not have more than $2,000 per month before taxes and income less than $1,869 per month in 2007. This figure changes every year to reflect the cost-of-living increase. It varies from state to state, too, so check with your state Medicaid office. This figure normally includes earned income such as wages, and unearned income such as interest and dividends. There are a few ways to proceed if your income is more than the requirement. Some states offer a Miller trust, a tool to handle excess money for those who do not receive enough monthly income to pay for nursing homes.

Income-cap states are states that will disqualify you from Medicaid if your income is $1 over the limit. A lawsuit has led to a solution to this problem. States are now allowed to set up a trust that pays the money to the nursing home, and Medicaid picks up the balance; this is called a qualified-income trust or Miller trust. A Miller trust allows a person medically cleared to enter a nursing home, but with too much income for Medicaid, to shelter this income into a trust. It is advisable to consult a lawyer to set up such a trust. This trust shelters only income, not assets.

A Miller trust allows income to be put into only the trust, not property. Income must be put into the trust during the month it is received and spent no later than the next month. You must put all the income from one source, such as Social Security or pension, into this trust. Sometimes you pay the nursing home a certain amount equal to the monthly balance, and then Medicaid pays the rest. Income in this trust does not count toward the income cap but does count toward co-payment for services.

For example, Jim has Social Security income of $1,700 and a pension of $400 per month. His income exceeds the limit of $2,000 by $100. A qualified income trust will be set up to receive the $2,100 that is paid over to the nursing home, and Medicaid will pay the balance of the bill. The nursing home bill is $4,000 per month, but Jim cannot pay this. The $2,100 will be put into trust and paid to the nursing home. Medicaid will pay the remaining $1,900.

Another way an applicant can meet the requirements if they have too much money is to "spend down" the income. Spend down means to reduce or bring down the asset/income to the appropriate level to qualify. Medical bills are subtracted from the income to help bring the individual's income in line with Medicaid requirements. Any mental or medical treatment counts toward spend down with Medicaid. This includes prescription drugs, emergency transportation, doctor visits, eyeglasses, hearing aids, durable medical equipment, psychologists, health-insurance premiums, and any expense that meets a medical need. The spend-down amount is the share of your income that is over the limit for Medicaid qualification.

A married couple has a more complicated set of rules to deal with to qualify for Medicaid than someone who is single. That is because each person's income can be treated as separate.

Another factor is that income is allowed for the person living at home to meet basic needs. The person living at home is called the community spouse. This does not affect the partner in the nursing home unless the spouse does not have enough to meet basic needs or has too many assets. The determining income is that of the partner who applies for Medicaid. Spouses are not held responsible for each other's long-term care. Expecting the well spouse to be totally responsible for the nursing home spouse would most likely put a dire financial strain on the community spouse's lifestyle. The cost of nursing homes can consume your savings in a few months.

If that person receives $500 from Social Security and $200 from a pension, that is the determining income toward the Medicaid limit.

If you own property jointly, any income that is generated will be divided 50/50. This applies to joint bank accounts, payments from a trust, or annuities. If you are living in the community or house, and your spouse is in the nursing home, you will not have to contribute any of your money to their care under Medicaid rules. The rules vary from state to state about what the community spouse is allowed to keep. Check with your state Medicaid agency.

MMMNA Explained

The community spouse is entitled to Minimum Monthly Maintenance Needs Allowance (MMMNA) to live in the house. The minimum varies, but for 2008 it is $1,711.25 per month, and the maximum is $2,610 per month. The monthly income allowance is the amount the nursing home spouse can contribute per month to the community spouse for living expenses. The amount that a community spouse is allowed to keep ranges from $104,400 to $20,000 annually, depending on the state. These ranges apply only if the community spouse needs the money to live in the community. Otherwise, the community spouse can use that income for his or her own expenses and needs.

This is how it works: Joe, who lives at home, gets only $700 a month from Social Security. His wife, who is in a nursing home, gets $2,000 a month — $1,000 from a teacher's pension and $1,000 from Social Security. Because the MMMNA is $1,711.25, the wife can give Joe $1,011.25 of her income to help him meet the minimum of allowance for the community spouse. The rest of her income can go to the nursing home, and Medicaid will pick up the balance of her bill.

The community spouse is allowed half of all joint countable assets. On average, the limit of income for the spouse in the nursing home is $2,000 per month. It is possible to increase the income of the community spouse above the minimum, allowing the couple to keep more of their assets and not give assets over to the nursing home. This can be done if shelter expenses for the community spouse exceed 30 percent of MMMNA. The shelter expenses include utilities, rent or mortgage, insurance, and taxes. This is called excess shelter allowance.

Another way to get some of the money shifted from the nursing home spouse to the community spouse is if the community spouse has family members living at home who are dependent, such as elderly parents or children. This creates a need for additional income in the household. In special cases where the maximum amount does not allow the community spouse to meet living expenses, you can ask for a fair hearing. A fair hearing is an appeal to Medicaid; it is a good idea to have an attorney help you with this matter. The laws have changed: Now the community spouse is allowed to keep more income, and the nursing home spouse does not give income to the community spouse unless there is a need.

Federal Spousal Impoverishment Act

The Federal Spousal Impoverishment Act, created in 1924, protects a person whose spouse enters a nursing home from losing all money and assets. The community spouse is allowed to keep enough income to live and run his or her home. When a spouse enters a nursing home, the nursing home should apply this law, especially if one person is still living at home. The community spouse needs to retain income to help with living expenses such as rent, food, medical, insurance, and other basic needs. This law applies when the spouse first enters the nursing home or applies for Medicaid.

Before someone goes into a nursing home, it is important to find out if the nursing home accepts Medicaid. Some nursing homes will not take Medicaid payments or accept people on the plan.

This law applies when one of the couple is expected to enter a nursing home for more than one month. The couple's resources when they apply for Medicaid are combined. The spousal share is usually half of the combined income or assets. The spousal share maximum was raised to $101,640 in 2007. A state can now set this amount between $20,000 and $101,640.

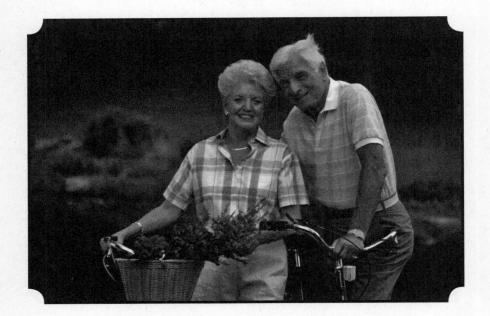

CHAPTER 2

Resources of the Single or Married Applicant

Determining Value of Assets

The value of an asset is the amount of money you can get for it in the marketplace, minus any debt. A home is a major asset. What you can sell a home for depends on the geographic region and the economy. A home worth $530,000 might sell for $550,000 if the market is right. Some assets are counted when determining Medicaid and others are excluded. Knowing the difference can help you act wisely with your assets.

Any asset that can be changed to cash is frequently considered a countable asset. A checking account, savings account, or cash in a vault in your house are all considered countable assets. Certificates of deposit, stocks, bonds, and mutual funds also are countable assets, as are IRAs and other kinds of retirement accounts, life insurance that can be converted to cash, annuities, and all autos except the first car. Extra buildings, machinery, and leisure items such as campers, boats, livestock, horses, and tractors may be countable assets.

Countable Assets

If you can spend it or convert it to cash, it is considered countable income under Medicaid.

Cash, checking accounts, savings and CDs (certificates of deposit) are countable income. Other investments, such as stocks and bonds, an IRA, 401k or other retirement account are all considered countable income. A life insurance cash value is countable if you can convert it to cash and the value is more than $1,500. If you own more than one car, the second, third, and fourth cars are countable. If you own more than one truck, tractor, boat, machinery, and livestock, those assets are countable. If you have additional land that is not excluded, it most likely is countable.

Bank deposits will regularly include savings, checking, CDs, or other accounts in a financial institution. An IRA is an individual retirement account that you maintain at a bank with special rules that allow you to avoid income tax until retirement. Tax laws impose heavy tax on early withdrawal of IRAs. It is undoubtedly a countable asset.

Securities include stocks, bonds, mutual funds, promissory notes, and other assets. A security is commonly countable unless it has no market value.

Excluded Assets

This may surprise you, but there are many assets that are excluded from Medicaid when determining eligibility. These assets are not countable toward your eligibility or your spouse's eligibility. The most basic rule, if you are single or married and determined eligible for Medicaid, is that you can have $2,000 cash — that is the limit. You have to keep your account below this or you can lose all Medicaid benefits.

Your home, if you are single and live in the house, is excluded from Medicaid if the equity is $750,000 or less. There are certain conditions that allow the home to be excluded if you are on Medicaid. One is if you will be in a nursing home for a certain period of time and plan to return. Another is if you have relatives who live in the house with you or own equity in the house — a spouse, dependent child, disabled child, sister or brother, or parents. The equity in the home is what Medicaid looks at. For instance, if you and your husband own a home worth $300,000, your equity in the house is $150,000.

If you are married and permanently in a nursing home, your home is excluded if your spouse or other relative live in the house. If you are in a nursing home and the value of your equity rises above the state limit, you can lose your Medicaid benefits. It is important to keep equity in the house below the limits set by Medicaid. The land the house sits on and other buildings are excluded as long as the equity is below $750,000.

Let us say that you live alone in the house and plan to return after your nursing home stay. You have been qualified for Medicaid to pay your nursing home expenses. If you are ill and cannot communicate your interest in returning to your house, a spouse or a dependent relative is allowed to communicate your intent to return to the house to a Medicaid or nursing home representative. If you moved from your home to an assisted living center or apartment, your home will not be excluded as an asset for Medicaid because it is not your main residence.

What about selling the house? The house is excluded as long as the money from the sale is used to purchase another home to live in no later than three months after the sale. Whatever money that is not invested into another home is counted. If your spouse lives in the house, the spouse can keep the money, as that person is considered the community spouse.

One auto is excluded, and it can be of any value. If the person owns more than one auto or other vehicles, those vehicles are countable at market value. If you own two cars, a motorcycle, and a truck, the second car, motorcycle, and truck, will be counted as assets.

Some personal property, such as jewelry, furniture, household appliances, and computers, are excluded from Medicaid, despite their value, if they are items used on a regular basis or items that have been in the family or hold sentimental value, such as wedding rings, necklaces, and artwork. Some items can be counted, especially if they are collected for investment purposes, such as jewelry, art, and other collectibles.

Funeral and burial expenses are often excluded, depending on the nature of the account. You can set aside about $1,500 in a bank account or trust for a funeral. This money will be excluded as long as it is below the limit and specified for this purpose. For a married couple, each person can have $1,500 in a bank account for funeral and burial expenses.

MassHealth allows four options for a prepaid funeral that is excluded. Cemetery plots may be purchased for a nursing home applicant, spouse, and any family members. A burial account may be started to pay for expenses not covered, with up to $1,500 each for husband and wife. You can buy a single premium insurance policy to pay for funeral expenses. Assigning the value of surrender to a funeral home makes the asset or value non-countable. Purchasing a prepaid funeral contract or irrevocable trust designated for funeral and burial expenses is an acceptable way to spend down assets. An irrevocable burial contract is not counted in Massachusetts.

Money people pay for their funeral and burial arrangements is excluded and no limit on the amount is set. You can spend as much as you want on your burial arrangements, even if you do it long before you become ill. If you make arrangements with a funeral home, the money you put aside must be put in an escrow account or trust. Some states require a contract declaring that any extra funds not used for funeral arrangements be paid to the nursing home or Medicaid. Even life insurance to be used for funerals or burials is excluded. You can prepay for burial expenses for your spouse and children, parents, and siblings. This includes burial spots, coffins, funeral proceeding, urns, and other traditional items.

If a Medicaid applicant is single, IRAs and other retirement accounts are countable assets. If an applicant is married and the spouse is living at home, these accounts often are not counted. Conversely, some states count the IRAs of both spouses.

Properties or buildings used for self-support by applicants normally are excluded from asset inclusion. If you own a small dairy farm that you make money from by selling milk, the farm property — including the land, buildings, and storage areas — is excluded. A small business at home used by you or your spouse may be excluded. Be aware that many states ignore this rule, or use the $6,000 or 6 percent rule. This means that if you own property not used in trade or business, but make money by renting it for use as a mobile home, only $6,000 of the property value can be excluded. This is especially true if you make a 6 percent or greater profit on renting land to mobile home users.

The life insurance policy owned by a Medicaid recipient frequently is excluded. The cash value of a policy smaller than $1,500 is not counted. If you want to keep a policy for burial, you might want to transfer the life insurance policy to a family member and have that person pay the premium if it helps with burial expenses.

Unavailable Assets

Some assets are not counted because they are not legally available to the person who is going on Medicaid. What circumstance determines whether an asset is unavailable? If a person does not have the legal right to use or dispose of an asset, that asset is considered unavailable. This can be because of a contract, court order, or law.

Assets that cannot be sold are unavailable. In order for an asset to be considered unavailable, you may have to produce evidence that it is not sellable. This can be done by getting experts in the geographic area with knowledge of assets to state in writing that the asset is not worth anything. For real estate, an actual sale attempt may have to be made to prove that it cannot be sold. If no offer is received, that is proof of it being unavailable.

If an asset is owned by more than one person and cannot be sold without the other person's consent, it is often unavailable. If the second person refuses to sell the asset, it is considered an unavailable asset.

If you are named an heir in someone's estate when they die, the inherited asset is not available to you until that person passes away. This asset would be excluded. If you own real estate that cannot be sold due to legal problems or other technical complications, this property would be excluded. A lawsuit that you filed prior to receiving Medicaid assistance where you were awarded money or that happened long before you filed for assistance would also be excluded.

What Are the 50 and 100 Percent States?

Some states allow the community spouse or person that is not in a nursing home to keep 50 percent of the couple's joint countable assets. This is especially true of married couples who have one person living in a nursing home due to chronic illness. These are known as the 50 percent states. Some states allow the community spouse to keep 100 percent of the couple's joint countable assets up to a certain dollar amount and not have to contribute the money to Medicaid. These are known as 100 percent states. Each state has different rules, so check with your state office.

The Snapshot Rule

The snapshot rule refers to the date an account of finances is looked at to see what should be counted or excluded, should an applicant eventually need Medicaid. It is normally the first day of the month a person enters the nursing home. The community spouse should get a resource assessment from a caseworker when a spouse enters a nursing home. This is not the same as applying for Medicaid, but will determine the couple's countable income. The sooner you get a resource assessment, the sooner you will know where your assets stand with social services.

Split Transfers

A split transfer offers the Medicaid applicant a method to shorten his or her eligibility period without having to give away all property before a 60-month look-back period. Under the 50/50 split transfer method, the person may give away half the property or assets during the look-back period and retain the other half. The gift is calculated as part of the ineligibility period. The person spends down the retained assets. Often, this cuts the ineligibility period in half. This is a conservative approach to save money on assets. One must plan ahead to do this successfully.

For example, John lives in a state where a nursing home cost $5,000 per month. He has $240,000 in assets. He gives his daughter $120,000 as a gift on June 1, 2006. He applies for Medicaid on May 1, 2010. The gift is within his 60-month look-back period, so he uses $120,000 for his nursing home care for this 12-month or longer ineligibility period.

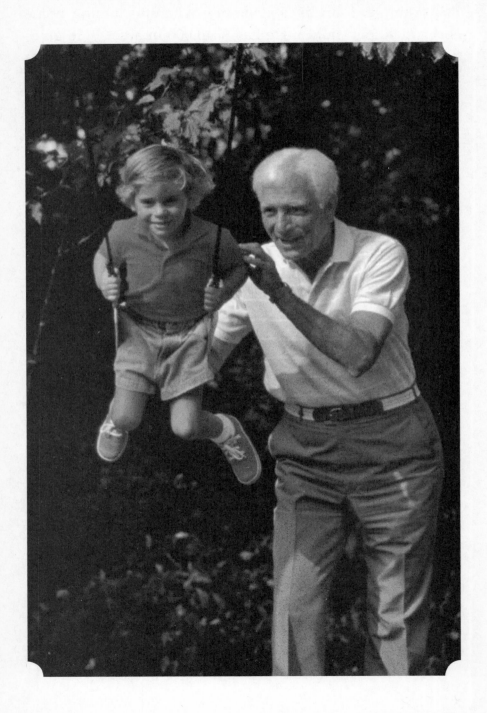

CHAPTER 3

Medicaid Estate Recovery

A Brief History of Estate Recovery

Most states recently have passed a law using estate recovery to help offset the growing financial burden of long-term healthcare using Medicaid. If someone is on Medicaid and that person dies, the state can go after assets that were previously excluded. If you own a house or if it has been passed to others in your family, the state can legally claim some of the assets to pay your Medicaid bill or your spouse's medical bill. This ruling varies from state to state.

Medicaid federal regulations now require this law of all states. Under many circumstances, the estate recovery law is waived in different states. The law is waived if there is a surviving spouse still living in the house or a spouse dependent on disabled children. If it causes hardship to the family, this regulation may be waived. If the person on Medicaid had a long-term health insurance policy that met with state requirements, this regulation often is used only for partial recovery. Each state will be given the ability to interpret and use this law for estate recovery.

For example, the state recovery unit may learn of the death of a person who was in a nursing home for five years on Medicaid. The state recovery unit will put in a claim against the member's probate estate, especially for unclaimed assets. Perhaps the person had a home that no one lives in; the state will try to get some of the equity from the home. Estate recovery claims in Massachusetts, for example, have increased yearly since 1999. The estate recovery laws have updated the definition of estate to include almost any asset the Medicaid recipient owns. It is important to know what is and what is not subject to estate recovery in your state. This is why it is imperative to work with an elder-care attorney who knows the latest laws.

There are always circumstances counted as exceptions to help prevent estate recovery. One is if you or the person in your family was under the age of 55, received Medicaid, and did not reside in a nursing home. If the Medicaid recipient is survived by a spouse living in the house, a child under the age of 21, or a dependent who is blind or permanently disabled as defined by Social Security rules, that person is not subject to estate recovery.

If a sibling or a son or daughter was living in the house one to two years before you entered the nursing home and continued to live there, you likely will not be subject to estate recovery. There are ways to object to estate recovery if it causes family hardship, such as leaving the family with nowhere to live or cutting off funds to meet living expenses.

Most states will file a claim within a year after the Medicaid recipient's death. If the state has a lien against the assets, it may have longer to file a claim on the asset or property. A family may not want to open a probate estate as a means to avoid the state's claim on the estate. Some states will file a claim as a creditor to open the probate estate when they find out that someone has died who was on Medicaid so they can collect the money the Medicaid recipient owes.

Liens on Your Estate or Home: How and Why?

A lien is a document filed by a creditor against your property or home that prevents the sale of your home or property without satisfying the debt owed. With the state Medicaid agency, a lien might be placed on the debt you or your family owes for medical coverage and nursing home care. States have the right to collect money that you owe for Medicaid recovery. A lien can be placed on a home once a recipient is expected not to return to that home. The lien can be filed if you are receiving nursing home services or HCBS. Liens may be placed against homes or land when you receive Medicaid benefits. Several years ago, Medicaid applicants were not allowed to own any property.

A lien cannot be filed if you have a spouse living in your house, a child who is under age 21, a disabled child as defined by Social Security, or a sibling who owns part of the house. The exception rule states that at least one to two years before you went into a nursing home, your children or brother or sister must have lived in the house and remained living there. The lien must be removed if you leave the nursing home and move back home.

The state of Massachusetts uses caseworkers to decide whether to use a living lien when a Medicaid applicant is approved.

If someone, such as a relative, is living in the house, a lien will usually not be put on the property; the property can be transferred without penalty at that time. If no one lives in the house, the caseworker must determine if the recipient will return home. If the recipient does not return home, no lien is put on the property, but the property is counted as an asset toward eligibility. This is waived for nine months, provided the member signs an agreement to sell the property for its fair market value. There are a few ways to release the lien when the property is sold, transferred, or refinanced. About 23 states now use liens for asset collection and estate recovery for Medicaid applicants using long-term care.

Medicaid Hardship Waivers

In some circumstances, the state might waive or not seek estate recovery. It might be because the money received would be small in relation to the amount of money used for recovery, or if recovery would cause undue hardship to the family for financial and other reasons.

A married couple should make plans that when one of them is on Medicaid, either person might become a survivor. When the spouse on Medicaid in a nursing home dies first, the state cannot recover any money if the community spouse still lives in the home and owns the other assets. If the community spouse dies before the spouse in a nursing home, you do not want the nursing home spouse to get the assets; he or she would then be disqualified from Medicaid. It is important to leave the house to children or other family members.

The state will not claim an estate if it is not cost-effective to do so. For instance, if the value of an estate is $10,000 or less, the cost of selling the property would be equal or greater than the value of recovery.

If the property or asset is used for a family business, a hardship waiver can be filed. You must prove the property or asset is used for income for family members and that a recovery claim would cause hardship. The asset must be a 50 percent or greater source of family income. An estate recovery claim can be rejected if the claim would force the family below the poverty level.

More About Medicaid Hardship Waivers

More states are going after the property of people on Medicaid than ever before as a way to recover the millions spent on long-term healthcare. Yet, there is a financial exception that allows individuals to get a hardship waiver. This is a way to get the state to lay aside claim on your family estate, especially if you had a family member on Medicaid in a nursing home for several years. The following exceptions are noted:

- Let us say a family member is exploited by someone in the family or a third party financially without knowledge, such as someone transferring assets so someone can qualify for Medicaid. If it is proved that the person did not know about this, a hardship waiver may be granted if assets cannot be returned.

- An eligibility worker can prove that denial of benefits will result in a life-threatening situation for the patient. All avenues including transfer penalty must be explored.

- If the person who received assets cannot be located and the ill person cannot return home to have care, that person might get a waiver. Or if physical harm will come to a patient by returning assets and that person has no place to return to, a waiver might be granted. If the receiver of the assets will not cooperate and has committed fraud, and the client has no place to return in the community, a waiver might be granted.

- An exception can be made if the power of attorney or person in charge transferred assets but did not act in the person's best interest, if the person was deprived of assets by fraud or misinterpretation, or if the person cannot recover the assets due to loss, destruction, or even theft.

- If the person who transferred assets made a reasonable effort to obtain return of assets, a waiver might be granted.

- A waiver might be granted if a client cannot access home equity in excess of $500,000 due to lien or legal problems and if, without these services, the client is in danger.

What Is a Survivorship Deed?

A survivorship deed is used when husband and wife purchase property together. It can also be used in other situations. This deed can allow owners to avoid probate upon one person's death, but when the second spouse dies, the property will be subject to probate. It is not suggested as a deed to be used between parents and children unless a lawyer is consulted first. If you want to divide the property equally among several people, this is the wrong deed to use. It can be used if a relative wants to name another co-owner of a home or property. If you have a deed made up long before you apply for Medicaid, the deed should not affect your eligibility. If you have a deed made up before you apply to avoid having your home or land factored in, that may count against you.

Other Deeds and Medicaid

Joint tenancy with rights of survivorship is a document or deed in which two people own half of the property equally. When one owner dies, the other acquires the right to the property completely; it is by right of survivorship. To establish ownership, the other party or survivor must get a certificate of death that is transferred out of probate, which makes it easy and profitable. The survivor is not required to record the deed, so it gives some privacy against parties who might object to the transfer. When one tenant or owner dies, creditors lose their rights against the property. It is an irrevocable deed and is taxable as a gift when it is executed.

An enhanced life estate deed is another name for a "Lady Bird" or joint tenancy deed. The owners retain the right to mortgage, sell, give a gift, or cancel the remaining interest at any time. Couples who want to attain full control over their property should use this type of deed.

It is a mistake to add children as survivors. If you deed property to children and retain life estate, your home may not be protected from creditors, and you may not qualify for Medicaid should you go into a nursing home. Your heir may have to pay a hefty gift tax on the property or assets. You may not be able to use your home to pay for the medical care you need.

The state of Massachusetts has a deed called a declaration of estate of homestead. It is filed with the Registry of Deeds in the county where your home or property is located and can protect property up to $500,000 of the value of a primary residence per family. A sole person commonly files this deed, and if family members own the house with you, they have homestead protection. It protects your home against attachment of levy or sale to satisfy debts. The property or home of persons 65 or older is protected and couples filing jointly will be protected despite martial status. A certified letter must be included when you register for declaration of estate of homestead by licensed physicians or the Social Security Administration. Only one spouse or person in the home under age 62 can file for this deed.

Liens imposed by the state for Medicaid are exempt from homestead protection. But the state will not file a suit especially if the spouse is alive. If the surviving spouse also is on Medicaid, the state will file a claim for reimbursement for the entire amount of Medicaid benefits paid. The rules are complicated, so it is good to get legal advice.

Estate Recovery Trends in Individual States

Michigan tends to ignore estate-recovery programs, much to the anger of taxpayers. The Deficit Reduction Act of 2005 enforces penalties on individuals who purposefully hide assets with the intention of qualifying for Medicaid. In Pennsylvania, estate means all property and all probate estate property; this means all real estate and personal property of the deceased person. Life insurance is subject to claim and also deposit and patient-care accounts.

States have different policies on estate recovery and some are more aggressive in seeking money from estates. Since Georgia instituted an estate-recovery program in May 2006, more than 100 patients have returned home or left the nursing homes they were in because of fear of losing their homes. Others have dropped Medicaid coverage or home-care services. Massachusetts has instituted a more aggressive program with liens against homes to claim an estate when a Medicaid recipient passes away.

Georgia and Michigan were the last two states to adopt estate recovery plans. This practice is causing heated debate because the state claims assets from estates of Medicaid applicants. Many live in nursing homes, then pass away owing Medicaid money. Many states have been slow to adopt the rules because it forces them to collect money from families that have used up money on long-term care. Some people feel this plan turns Medicaid into a predatory loan for those over 55.

States with limited budgets seek to recover some of the money lost on the Medicaid program. The goal of Medicaid estate recovery is not to bankrupt people but to receive some money back.

Utah recovers money from the estate of Medicaid recipients providing there is no heir who is blind, disabled, or under the age of 21. Recovery takes place only after the death of the Medicaid recipient and the surviving spouse. The maximum amount of recovery is the amount paid for medical expenses for a recipient age 56 and older. Your home is exempt for Medicaid eligibility but not from estate recovery.

Utah proceeds with estate recovery by having the Office of Recovery Services contact the heirs after the death of the Medicaid recipient. The organization may record a lien against real property of a deceased recipient to obtain estate recovery. They may file a claim with the court for the amount of medical assistance provided.

Florida estate recovery will not file a claim if there is a surviving spouse, if the recipient is under the age of 55, or if a minor or disabled child lives in the estate. The state only claims the amount paid on behalf of the Medicaid recipient for services rendered.

Florida law requires any representative of an estate to notify all creditors. Medicaid is considered a creditor of an individual receiving benefits from the Medicaid program. State agencies such as the Vital Statistics and Social Security offices often share information about deaths of Medicaid recipients with state agencies. This is the way the states know to file a claim on a Medicaid applicant's estate.

In Indiana, when a Medicaid recipient dies or has an estate, a claim will be filed against the estate for reimbursement for services paid on behalf of that person when they are age 65 or older. This includes services to those under 55 if made after October 1, 1993. Claims include all services provided to Medicaid recipients.

All assets are subject to estate recovery. Many assets not counted for Medicaid eligibility may be counted in estate recovery. Assets not subject to recovery are life insurance or annuities. The first $125,000 of jointly held property with right of survivorship in Indiana is not subject to estate recovery. Real estate used for the support of a surviving spouse is excluded. Personal effects, keepsakes, and ornaments of the deceased are other items often excluded.

The state of Virginia asked the U. S. Court of Appeals to approve an exemption that would allow homeowners to retain $50,000 of their home against Medicaid claims to recover the cost of nursing home care; federal Medicaid officials denied the request in 2007. Many West Virginians refuse to apply for Medicaid due to the new rulings.

In Pennsylvania, Medicaid applicants are often told about the estate recovery program by caseworkers during the application process. Only medical assistance received after the age of 55 and for specific types of services are subject to estate recovery. The state seeks reimbursement for nursing facilities, home and community, and hospital and prescription drug services.

New York requires recovery from the estate of Medicaid recipients who are 55 or older. It can recover from the estate of the spouse except if the spouse is still living in the house or has a disabled child under 21 living in house. The state filed a claim against a couple's estate both deceased for $386,327.77. The man had left a supplemental needs trust for $15,000 for his mentally retarded son. In this case, because the husband was found responsible for his wife's care by the state, the state decided the trust to his son was a countable asset for estate recovery.

Oregon has tough new Medicaid estate recovery policies for long-term care. The new rules can collect money from your estate after you die for Medicaid costs, for long-term care in a nursing home, or for home services. A nursing home spouse used to be able to transfer the house to the well spouse to shield the assets from Medicaid use. Now, if someone transfers the house within the five-year look-back period, the house becomes a countable asset. It will be hard for people to protect their homes from estate recovery if they need Medicaid in the future.

CHAPTER 4

Asset Protection Strategies

Transferring Assets: Tips for Doing It the Right Way

The Medicaid look-back period changed in 2006 from three years to five years. It starts with the date of the transfer of assets to the date the individual goes into the nursing home and applies for Medicaid. The penalty period does not begin until the person is out of funds. Influencing these changes is the Deficit Reduction Act of 2005, which states that anyone with home equity over $500,000 is ineligible for Medicaid. This act requires a new way to deal with annuities, requiring the state be named as remainder beneficiary. This act allows continuing-care communities to spend down resources before applying for medical assistance. All states must apply the income-first rule to the community spouse. It extends the long-term care partnership to any state requesting that they be part of this program.

The look-back period discourages any gift giving by anyone who may need long-term care or has the possibility of needing it. It prohibits Medicaid for anyone who has home equity in excess of $500,000. Some states may increase this to $750,000. Anyone with equity above the limit will have to sell his or her home to get Medicaid. Transfers made five years before application for Medicaid are not penalized. The funds should be held in trusts for entire family benefit. Long-term care insurance purchase is encouraged as a way to offset costs.

The universal rule is that the value of any gift is the market value. It should be sold to the common public for a retail price. This also applies to bank accounts, counting the value of what you get when you liquidate the account. Life insurance cash value is what is counted — ignore term life insurance. Real estate sometimes requires an appraisal.

Trusts and Medicaid

The purpose of a trust is to protect, manage, and hold assets for your family or heir. Someone must make the trust specify who, what, when, where, and why. The trust should specify how property should be invested. If the contract is written for the benefit of someone such as an elderly person, making the trustee a family member, friend, or heir is practical. A revocable trust is when properties or assets are transferred from one person to another.

There are three elements to a trust document. The grantor is the person with the money who owns the trust. The grantor wants to get assets out of his or her name to prevent lawsuits and for asset protection. The trustee is the person who manages the trust. Beneficiaries are the family members, friends or associates, or charitable organizations you leave assets to. Before you implement any trust, know the pros and cons of having one. The advantages of most trusts are asset protection, tax planning, avoiding expense, delay of probate, confidentiality, estate planning, and gaining flexibility.

The Miller trust only solves one problem — if the person applying has too much income and/or assets to qualify for Medicaid. Other names for this trust are income-cap or income-assignment trust. The person who creates the trust assigns the right to receive Social Security and pension to the trust. Thus, the trust is receiving the income, not the person.

If the person is going to receive care at home, he or she should not give all the income to the Miller trust, but just part of the income. For example, if a man receives $900 from Social Security and $600 from his pension, he should assign only his Social Security to it; whatever it takes to get the income level down for Medicaid. A power of attorney can create a Miller trust for a disabled person. You then create a bank account for the trust. The bank account cannot have an opening balance. Then, you write to your Social Security or pension office and have them deposit funds to this trust. This is not a long-range planning tool, but for someone who plans to apply for Medicaid in the next few months.

If you have a will and disinherit family members, your will may be an open invitation to lawsuits. If you have a missing heir, that heir may be notified of the pending probate that could result in your estate being tied up for years. A trust avoids probate and your assets will be distributed to whom you specified by the trustee.

Revocable Living Trusts

This is used for married couples in Medicaid planning. It is not that helpful to a single person seeking Medicaid assistance. A revocable living trust aims to increase the amount that the community spouse or person not going into a nursing home is allowed to keep. The property loses its exempt status; this will help the community spouse get half of the assets when counted. You can sometimes spend down the trust by transferring the property out of the trust into the ownership of the community spouse. If one person owns the trust, it will be counted by the state for Medicaid purposes.

The revocable trust does not protect your assets from lawsuit, or estate taxes. Because the person that grants the trust is normally the trustee, he still owns money or assets and is subject to claims against it. The best it does is eliminate probate, serving as an extension of your will.

Actually, it is a popular alternative to a will as a way to pass property on after you die. It is made for management and fair distribution of your property. It can be changed or eliminated at any time because it is revocable. The trusts are established by written agreement and appointment of a trustee to manage the property. The trust gives detailed instructions that tell how the property will be managed and distributed.

Any competent adult can establish a revocable trust. Husbands and wives often establish a trust together. It can instruct that their community and separate property assets be held in different accounts. A revocable trust avoids probate because you collect your assets and transfer them to the trustee before you die. It does not avoid estate, income, and gift taxes. A federal estate tax return must be filed after you die if your net is worth more than 1.5 million dollars.

The trust should own the title or property to which it belongs. Transferring assets or title is called funding the trust. The trust has a grantor or person who sets up the trust. They have the power to change or control the trust at any time. The trustees are the person or persons who will manage the trust. Sometimes the grantor and trustee are the same person. You need to name a successor trustee, a person who manages the trust when you die. The person will have the same power as the grantor after he passes away. This person does not have the legal right to change your trust. It becomes irrevocable or unchangeable after the grantor dies.

Grantor Irrevocable Trust

A person who could utilize this trust is someone living in an assisted living center. They need a personal attendant to live in the assisted living center or be in a nursing home. Medicaid does not pay for companion care.

The trust would be used so the assets are not counted when a person applies for Medicaid. They can make the gift without a trust. There are more risks making an outright gift. This includes the fact that the creditor may attach the gift or seek money from the gift so that it benefits neither the giver nor the person receiving it. The child's spouse can make a claim against the gift in a divorce; the person receiving the gift becomes disabled so it is used for their medical problems. The elderly person can even be trustee to this trust.

This trust addresses these risks. The adult creates the trust and funds it with assets, such as a house, cash, or securities. Money can still be used for the adult and the person can even be the trustee. It can result in a penalty against anyone applying for Medicaid assistance. If an adult is using cash and securities for income, this money can still be used to assist them.

The grantor is the person with the money or owner of the assets. The trust specifies that this has to be an adult not entitled to receive the principal distribution from the trust. This means the adult is severing his or her ties from the assets. The trust also has a spendthrift clause that specifies that the principal is unavailable to the child's creditors. It can hold assets for the child even after the adult dies. It has three elements: grantor, trustee, and beneficiaries. The trustee is the person who is empowered to carry out the terms of the trust agreements. When asset protection is important, the trustee should not be the same person as the grantor. The beneficiaries are the persons who will benefit from the income or assets of the trust.

A transfer of the house or other assets to the grantor can be advantageous. Capital gains taxes can be wiped out on the death of the elderly person who makes the trust. He or she can maintain the trust while making plans to pass it on after his or her death or disability.

Under 65 Payback Trust

Sometimes, a person under 65 years old needs care in a nursing home, or the person needs to be eligible for medical care insurance for long-term care. A person with too many resources can gift his or her assets to this trust. Congress created the rules for this trust for a person under the age of 65. The trustee can use the assets within the trust. When the person dies, the fund must first be applied to reimburse the state, especially if the person was on Medicaid. The rest can go to the family members it was left to. When someone transfers assets or money to this trust, it does not normally penalize him or her for applying for Medicaid. The patient or conservator can create it.

Rules make it more advantageous for persons under 65 to create a special needs trust, which allows some exceptions for a trust established by a parent, grandparent, guardian or conservator. The beneficiary must be disabled as defined by the Social Security Act. If the beneficiary is receiving SSD (Social Security Disability) or SSI (Supplemental Security Income) the requirement is met. At the death of the beneficiary, the remaining payback trust balance must be given to Medicaid.

The establishment of the trust depends on whether the person who needs it has parents or grandparents to make decisions. If the person does not, a court will appoint someone to make decisions for them.

A Medicaid payback trust is established to prevent the funds from an estate or personal injury suit from disqualifying an older or younger disabled person from benefits like Social Security and Medicaid. Trust money may be useful for many medical and personal services not covered by Medicaid.

Testamentary Supplemental-Needs Trust

This is used when a married couple has one person on Medicaid. If the community spouse dies, the assets should not go to the nursing home spouse. This would give the nursing home spouse too many resources and would disqualify them from Medicaid. The attorney writes a will that disinherits the nursing home spouse. In most states, you cannot disinherit a spouse completely. In Arizona, for example, if a spouse is disinherited, the law says they are entitled to receive allowances and exemptions up to $37,000. If the nursing home spouse does not exercise the right to receive this, the state may disqualify them from Medicaid for ten months or more; this trust addresses this problem. The community spouse creates a will giving all assets to children except for the $37,000 special needs trust in favor of the nursing home. Because the funds are in a special trust, they do not count against the nursing home spouse. It will not disqualify them from Medicaid and can be used to purchase items that Medicaid does not purchase, such as dental work, furniture, TV, and companion care. This trust can also work for a disabled person without jeopardizing the disabled person's eligibility. A family could set up this trust for a disabled elderly relative, and that would not disqualify them from Medicaid.

This trust is designed to preserve SSI, Medicaid, and other public assistance benefits when unexpected events occur. For instance, when an adult in a nursing home receives public benefits and is awarded an inheritance. Or when a disabled adult in a nursing facility receives proceeds from a personal injury settlement or suit. This trust will set up the money to be used for other medical and personal care needs not covered by Medicaid or public assistance.

Other supplemental needs not covered are alternative medical therapies, physician specialists not covered by Medicaid, massage sessions, haircut and salon services, over-the-counter medications such as vitamins and herbs, personal assistance, taxi rides, travel expenses to visit family, furniture, clothing, cell phones, vacation trips, attorney fees, and more.

This trust allows a disabled person to maintain eligibility for government benefits such as Medicaid and supplemental security income.

Revocable and Irrevocable Trusts: What They Are and What They Do

A trust is a document with a set of specific instructions to a person called a trustee. It is a legal document enforceable by law. The issues addressed by trusts include: how the person's assets will be used; who gets the assets when the trust ends or the person dies; what debts and taxes can be paid with the trust; who the trustees are; what power the trustees have with the assets; and how can the assets be invested.

Trusts are useful if you are leaving money to people who would spend it before they receive it. A trust protects your beneficiary from other family members who might go after the money or trick others out of the money they deserve. A trust is useful to plan for your own disability or long-term health concerns.

A trust allows a person to manage property or assets for the benefit of another person. Trust property can be many different types of assets, such as cash, stocks, real estate, and CDs. The property in the trust is called the principal of the trust. Interest or revenue generated by the trust is called the trust income.

Revocable Trusts

A revocable trust, also called a living trust, is a trust that can be changed by creators at any time. These are not recommended for Medicaid planning. Since the person can change the trust anytime, all assets are considered countable toward Medicaid eligibility.

Revocable trusts are useful for estate planning. These trusts can help you avoid probate, manage your assets, and provide privacy. Be leery of anyone claiming a living trust to protect you from a Medicaid claim or help you become eligible should you need long-term care. Assets in this trust are all countable assets.

Irrevocable Trusts

An irrevocable trust is a trust that cannot be changed or revoked by the person who creates it. These trusts are useful for Medicaid planning purposes. If the transfer to the trust is considered a gift, it is no longer a countable asset. Once the Medicaid look-back period or penalty period expires, the trust is ignored. For example, if you transfer all your assets into the right irrevocable trust, wait five years and apply for Medicaid, the trust would not be counted. That is an ideal situation that you cannot count on.

An income-only irrevocable trust is a trust used specifically for Medicaid. Medicaid considers the assets of this trust not countable. The person who makes the trust gives up all rights to the principal assets of the trust, but has the right to all income generated by those assets. If, for example, real estate, such as home and land, is involved in a trust, often the person can live in the house. This trust provides the flexibility to sell assets such as real estate, while protecting principal assets.

Irrevocable trusts do not give you the flexibility to change your mind. Once the assets are transferred, you cannot get them back. Your use of the trust is restricted forever — you cannot use money for a trip or to pay your nursing home bill. You get the guarantee that your heir will get the asset or property. It will not be sold or claimed by the state to pay for the nursing home bill. A transfer to this deed disqualifies you from Medicaid for five years, so this method should not be used if you expect to enter a claim before that.

Irrevocable trusts protect assets because the grantor transfers assets to an independent trustee. Because the person does not own the trust, it is not subject to taxes. The assets can be deferred from capital gains taxes.

Self-Settled and Pooled Trusts

Another trust worth discussing is a self-settled trust, which is a trust created for your own benefit. It protects your assets from creditors and others who may try to get the money or property, yet are not entitled to it. Sometimes, these trusts are self-settled spendthrift trusts. In the 1990s, these trusts became popular. Many states do not recognize this trust, but if you are under the age of 65 and disabled, a trust such as this can be established for you. Your assets will not be counted by Medicaid. Such trusts must be established by a parent, grandparent, legal guardian, or court. You must have a payback clause that states you will repay Medicaid all debts owed through the state. Such trusts can supplement what Medicaid pays for, and will leave some assets to family instead of the state.

Pooled trusts under current laws will be counted against those on pubic assistance, so this type of trust would cut off or disqualify an applicant from Medicaid. It is also a trust set up by a nonprofit organization in a state that holds funds of disabled individuals to be used to supplement their income. In this case, Medicaid would not count the trust. Contributions from each person are counted separately, but all money collected is pooled as one source to be used for the group. If a person is under 65, he or she is not penalized, but some states view pooled trusts as countable for persons over 65. Money can be used for items that Medicaid does not pay for.

Pooled trusts benefit the elderly person who is infirm and some nursing home residents and recipients of government assistance programs. It can be used for elderly care services, guardian fees, supplemental nursing care, and medical procedures not covered by government care. Other needs, such as clothing, medical insurance, handicapped vans, vacations, and travel expenses are included.

Irrevocable Life Insurance Trust Pros and Cons

These trusts hold your life insurance policy, removing it from your estate. Once it is created, it cannot be changed. So once you place the insurance policy in another person's name, you cannot take it back under your own name. You can control who your beneficiaries of the policy will be. You also can define the way they receive benefits.

You can choose who will be your trustee. It is important to get good legal advice to set this up properly because it undoubtedly will give you tax breaks.

Some people feel these trusts are too complicated and expensive to maintain. They are not worth the potential tax savings for some. You lose the ability to use the cash value of the policy, should you change your mind and want to cash it in. If your circumstances change, you cannot alter this type of trust.

The premiums are frequently paid by annual gifts made to the trust by the person who established it. The trustee cannot be trust originator, but might be someone from your bank or an accountant. Due to the complexity of this type of trust, you may want to use someone who is a professional.

You set the terms of the asset distribution in this trust. You can have assets distributed in total to all your beneficiaries immediately, or you can arrange to have certain members receive monthly or periodic distributions from the trust. You can dictate that someone must be at least 25 years of age before they receive any money. You can use this trust to help someone with educational costs or a business start-up. Most people name their children and grandchildren as beneficiaries. A trustee will follow your direction on how to use this trust and will pay your insurance premiums and file a tax return.

You can use an individual life insurance policy or, if your spouse is alive, you can use a survivorship policy. This pays out death benefits after both spouses pass away. You cannot stop your beneficiaries from withdrawing money from the trust, so it is important to have their cooperation for this policy. If you decide you do not want to continue to pay the premiums, a way to get rid of this policy is by letting it lapse.

This trust works well by taking advantage of the tax break called annual gift tax exclusion. You need to send your beneficiaries notice of what you have done to qualify for this gift tax. You can apply your annual insurance premium toward this gift tax. In a 1968 court battle, Dr. Clifford Crummey challenged the IRS and won the right to apply his insurance premium toward the gift tax inclusion.

When you own a regular life insurance policy when you die, the insurance proceeds are subject to taxes. For example, Joe Smith, a widower, has an estate worth $3 million. The estimated taxes on his estate are $675,000. He takes out a $1 million policy to pay the taxes. He owns the insurance policy. When he dies, the policy is subject to taxes of 45 to 47 percent, or $470,000 of policy pay estate tax. One way around this is for him not to own a policy when he dies. If someone else owns it, then it is not taxable. The primary benefit of this policy is that taxes are saved.

The trustee can purchase a life insurance contract on your life with funds that you provide. If you transfer an existing policy and die three years after transfer, it will be included in your estate. Sometimes, conditions are imposed when you transfer a policy. A taxpayer can give $11,000 to another person as a gift tax-free. This can buy lots of life insurance.

The trustee will pay the annual life insurance premium. The trustee must notify the beneficiaries in writing that a gift has been made in their name. Your beneficiaries will have the option of withdrawing funds in 30 days, on average. Written notification of your gift to beneficiaries is the so-called Crummey letter. An annual Crummey letter is an essential element of the irrevocable life insurance trust.

Charitable Remainder Trusts

Charitable remainder trusts serve two purposes: they help the disadvantaged and help the wealthy reduce their tax bills.

In 1969, Congress created a bill to help charities increase the revenues for their causes. The trust allows taxpayers to reduce estate taxes, eliminate capital gains, claim an income tax deduction, and benefit nonprofit organizations. This trust is called a charitable remainder trust.

These trusts are irrevocable trusts that provide for two sets of beneficiaries. The first set is the income beneficiaries, which can be you and your spouse if you are married. The income beneficiaries receive a set percentage of income for life from the trust. The second set of beneficiaries is the charities or nonprofit organizations you name. They receive the principal of the trust after the beneficiaries pass away. Even though this trust is irrevocable, you can change the charitable beneficiaries at any time. In certain cases, you can serve as trustee and retain control of all assets inside the trust.

Because the assets are for a charity, you do not pay any capital gains tax on this trust. These taxes can range from 10 to 20 percent on the asset's growth. This is ideal for stocks or property with low-cost basis but high appreciated value. It allows you to sell your assets without the tax which passes at full value to trust and family members. The amount of income depends on the percentage of payout you choose and the amount of income the assets generate. The IRS states that the trust must distribute about five percent of market value of assets to be a valid account.

Many people use this trust to help with retirement planning. By setting one up in peak earning years you can contribute in a variety of ways like zero coupon bonds, non-dividend paying growth stocks, or variable annuities. By letting it grow and not using money, you can have income when you retire — no limit on how much you can contribute. It is considered outside your estate by the IRS; due to this you can save 48 cents on every dollar. Because these accounts benefit a charity, they qualify you for an income tax deduction. Average deductions range from 20 to 50 percent against your gross income.

529 Plans and Medicaid: How They Work

Medicaid counts 529 plans as assets, making them a less desirable plan. If your grandparents saved money in a 529 plan for your college education, that was incredibly admirable. On the other hand, if your grandmother goes into a nursing home and goes on Medicaid or needs to qualify, this account will be counted and used by the state for payment. If you are the granddaughter and you counted on that $60,000 for paying for your college education, you might be in for a letdown. It might be wise to try to find other ways to finance your education. That is the downside of this plan; it is an educational savings plan operated by the state or educational institution. This is considered a gift, so that is why it will be counted if you need Medicaid assistance.

Some states with Medicaid are excusing this plan or making it exempt. One state that has done this is Arkansas. On, March 29, 2007, a bill was signed into law in Arkansas called Bill 822. It specifies that the 529 savings plans will be exempt for purposes of determining eligibility for Medicaid, food stamps and other government assistance. This is provided the federal rule permits an exemption. Other states should follow this example and make the plan exempt. Until all states make this account exempt, consider keeping the account out of your name. Your best bet is to make contributions through the 529 plan and have the plan owned by your grandchildren's parents. You can establish a custodial plan that transfers direct ownership to the beneficiary at age 18 or 21.

A new method is called a 529 savings plan. You should keep the 529 savings plan out of the name of anyone applying or needing Medicaid. The account should be in the name of younger, healthier relatives. Your children or grandchildren might be a good choice to transfer the plan to. That way, you will not have it counted when and if you need Medicaid.

What If Someone Contests the Trust?

The law in many states treats trusts like wills, so they are taken seriously. They can be contested if it is proven that someone who did not have the mental capacity to make a trust was under forceful influence. A trust is more likely to be challenged than a will because it is specific and the rules must be followed. Those who are not beneficiaries have no right to see a copy of the trust.

Why Are Trusts Better Than Outright Gifts?

Trusts protect your assets from your creditors and children while you are alive. An outright gift is open season for anyone to try to get a piece of the action. With a trust, you can serve as trustee with your family named as successors; then you can control and invest assets as you see fit. Once you give it away, you lose control and the person who has it may spend it all that same day. Trust assets will not count against you should you need to apply to Medicaid. The state cannot go after your trust assets after you die to try to recover the money paid for your medical treatment.

A trust protects assets from claims should your children get divorced. A gift is often spent or out of your control once it is given. It saves income tax for your children and permits income to be distributed to you for life. It permits backdoor distribution to members of your family should that ever be a necessity. A trust does not increase the Medicaid look-back period as an outright gift does. Previously, gifts were better than trusts, but now the law proves the opposite.

The drawback is that trusts cost money to prepare, as they can cost from $1,000 to $2,500 in preparation fees. It takes time to understand exactly how they work. You will have to open a separate bank account for the trust. You will have to have a federal ID number for the trust. A separate income tax must be filed each year.

Advanced Directives

Advanced directives are written oral statements about how you want medical decisions followed should you become ill and not able to make decisions for yourself. These are directed to your doctor and healthcare providers. They can express your wish to donate an organ after death. Some people make these after recovering from a life-threatening illness or as part of their estate that they plan to leave to relatives. There are many forms of advanced directives. They vary from state to state.

Advanced directives allow you to appoint someone to make your healthcare decisions. Older persons may want to think about having them as they age. All 50 states have laws regarding advanced directives. You can revoke or withdraw the advanced directives at any time. Some states have advanced directives for mental health treatments and physical illnesses.

The drawback of advanced directives is that often doctors do not notice them, even if the directives are placed in the patient's chart. Sometimes, the documents are written with terms that are ambiguous or difficult to apply. Physicians may disagree on what "terminally ill" means. Physicians might also ignore these documents due to pressure from family or belief that another treatment may help the patient. Some physicians may fear they would be sued if they withheld life support. A living will and medical power of attorney are two main forms of advanced directives.

A Living Will

A living will is a written oral statement of medical care about what you specifically want and do not want when you become unable to take care of yourself and make decisions. It is called a living will because it takes effect while you are still living. A healthcare provider or good attorney can help you prepare this document. It is important because it will help you control what you want to happen when you are ill and cannot speak for yourself. This may never happen, but it is good to be prepared.

Do not confuse this with a living trust, which is used to hold and distribute a person's assets. A living trust is used to avoid probate. A living will varies from state to state, so you may want to have a lawyer prepare yours. Many lawyers who practice estate planning provide a living will and healthcare power of attorney preparation in one complete package.

You may want to talk with your doctor about the type of medical treatments you would refuse if you were in a coma or vegetative state. He or she can answer any questions you may have about these medical procedures.

Living wills by and large describe life-prolonging treatments that you and the doctor may not not want to use. This is in the event you suffer a terminal illness or are in a vegetative state. It only becomes effective when you no longer are able to speak for yourself. Certification by your doctor and another medical person would have to be made in many cases for you to use it.

Be sure to talk with your doctor and the person you put in charge of your living will. Keep it in a place where you know it is safe but accessible for others in the event they need a copy.

Draft a living will with a lawyer specializing in elder law because it is a complex document that needs someone who understands the law. Your signature and a few witnesses are normally a standard requirement for a living will. In some states, your signature must be notarized to make the will legal. Some states do not allow you to use your doctor or relatives as witnesses.

Once the will is completed, give a copy to your doctor, family members, a member of your religious community, the hospital you use, and the nursing home if you live at one.

Below is an example of a situation that requires a living will. Bob was 65 when he had a fatal heart attack at home. He was rushed to the hospital and hooked up to a machine. He was in a vegetative state but kept alive by these machines. His wife Mary wanted him disconnected, but his parents wanted him to stay on life support because they believed he would eventually get better. He never made out a will, so no decision could be made for him by any family member. He was unable to make any decisions, so this left everyone in a limbo about how to proceed. Needless to say, the cost of his care escalated and the fight whether or not to keep him alive caused family members unnecessary stress. If he had a living will made, this would have helped the situation.

If you were in a nursing home permanently and suffered from a stroke after age 65, a living will would give someone you trust the power to do what you want with your healthcare. You might be sent to the hospital and hooked up to a life support machine even if they could not save you. If you have no living will, the system can drain your finances and control your fate. A living will is a good idea for anyone concerned about the big picture with healthcare. It gives someone you trust the power to make decisions for you when you no longer can.

A Healthcare Surrogate Designation

A healthcare surrogate designation, similar to a living will, is a document naming another person as your representative to make medical decisions for you if you are unable to make them for yourself. This can include instructions about any treatment you do not want.

Any competent adult can be named your surrogate, who can make healthcare decisions for you during time of incapacity; they should consult with your healthcare providers. They only make decisions for the person who made the living will. The decisions are based on what the person directed them to do or would have done themselves if they could. You can designate an alternative surrogate in case the primary surrogate is unable or unwilling to assume the responsibility. A copy must be provided to the healthcare surrogate and unless a termination date is given, this will remain in effect until the person with the living will revokes it.

The living will and healthcare surrogate can be revoked at any time using a signed and dated letter from the maker. It is important to tell your physician that the living will and surrogate have been revoked. For instance, you can direct the person to donate your organs after death or not to allow you to be kept alive by life support if you are technically dead.

An anatomical donation is when you allow donations of all or part of your body upon death. This can be organs and tissue donated to persons in need or donated to a healthcare facility for training purposes for doctors and interns. Organ donors can donate through driver's license renewal or state ID application, or you can put it in a living will.

When planning or making advanced directives, you should ask surrogates if they agree to be responsible for your health decisions, and give them a copy after they sign the legal documents. They should know where the documents are located should they need them. You also can use an attorney to do this.

Set up a file for advanced directives and paperwork. Some people keep them in a bank safety-deposit box. You can keep a card or note in your purse or wallet with information on the safety-deposit box.

Durable Power of Attorney

A durable power of attorney for healthcare is another form of advanced directive. It designates a person you have chosen to make healthcare decisions. It becomes active any time you become unable to make decisions for yourself. The person must be 18 years or older to be an advocate for your healthcare needs. You can pick a family member or friend to be your representative. It can be used to accept or refuse medical treatment. Sometimes, your lawyer serves as durable power of attorney.

A nondurable power of attorney is used for specific transactions like closing on the sale of a house. It is frequently used to handle a person's financial matters. Another form of this is called the springing power of attorney. This is used for future events, like an illness or disability of the principal. It requires a doctor to determine that the person is not competent to handle his or her financial affairs. It remains in effect unless revoked by a court.

Durable and springing powers of attorney are often used for planning for someone's healthcare needs. For example, if a person were to get Alzheimer's disease or suffer a severe handicap, it would help them manage their financial affairs.

Someone who has the power of attorney can buy or sell your real estate, manage your property, conduct your banking transactions, invest or not invest your money, make legal claims, attend to tax and retirement matters, and make gifts on your behalf.

Different States and Advanced Directives

Arizona has three types of medical will power of attorney: healthcare power of attorney, a living will, and a pre-hospital medical care directive. California has a healthcare agent, a person with the power to discharge or hire healthcare providers, refuse or consent to treatment, or withhold or sustain life-sustaining treatment. These people do not have power over your financial life. In Connecticut, a living will is mentioned. This is a will that gives specific instructions about medical treatment should you become ill or unable to make decisions, or express an interest in donating body organs for research or transplant. There are specific forms for all these legal directives to fill out. When filling out these forms, consult an attorney who is familiar with the laws concerning the elderly, including recent changes in the law.

CHAPTER 5

Annuities

What Are Annuities?

Annuities are comparable to insurance policies. You pay a monthly premium like an insurance policy. An annuity is a popular type of investment for people to make because the investment will grow on a tax-deferred basis. The owner of the annuity has the right to change the beneficiary of the annuity. The annuitant is the person whose life expectancy the payment is based on.

With a Medicaid annuity, the beneficiaries receive payment only if there is a guarantee period specified in the policy and the annuitant dies before the end of his or her life expectancy. The guarantee period is the length of time the payments for the annuity will be made. It often will terminate on death of the person. The guarantee period helps if the person who owns the policy dies in two years, and payments will continue if the policy was purchased for more years. For example, if the person purchased a ten-year guarantee period and died in two years, the payments will continue for eight years. This means beneficiaries of the policy will continue to get payments for eight years and payments will not stop with the annuitant's death. A guarantee period is important with an annuity for

Medicaid or other purposes. It must be purchased with this guarantee as part of the terms.

Another definition of an annuity is a savings plan used by individuals for long-term growth and savings. It protects their assets and will be used for retirement. Many use these every year to guarantee asset protection and to have a nest egg to fall back on. It can provide tax-preferred benefits, long-term growth, interest rates, probate protection, and lifetime income. Insurance companies provide most annuity products.

Another reason annuities are popular is that they are not taxed immediately and often do not drop below the value or price you paid for the annuity. The owner of the annuity has a right to change the beneficiary. A guarantee period clause should be included to ensure annuity payment will be made, even if the person the policy was taken out for dies. The annuity terminates on death of the annuitant without this clause.

Medicaid Annuities

A Medicaid Annuity is an annuity used to protect your assets immediately from the cost of long-term medical care such as nursing homes. Since Medicaid does not pay nursing home costs if you have too many assets, many people with liquid assets more than $2,000 are using this technique. A person transfers assets to a third-party insurance company to purchase an annuity that guarantees the owner a fixed monthly income for life.

Some states disapprove of this tactic, but many states have a policy for this procedure. The annuity contract must be irrevocable, non-transferable and have equal payments over the lifetime of the annuity. Since payments are fixed, you will receive a check for the same amount every month regardless of the performance of the stock market. You cannot withdraw the principal of the annuity once purchased. In some cases, the annuity may be put in the community spouse's name if the other spouse has plans to enter a nursing home.

The Deficit Reduction Act of 2005 now has a new rule on annuities. Any purchased after this date must name the state as a beneficiary in order not to have the annuity counted as an asset when applying for Medicaid. This is the only way to purchase an annuity and not have it counted for Medicaid if you became ill and had to get long-term assistance.

Annuities and Medicaid

An annuity is a great way to plan for medical assistance because once you buy an annuity, it is not counted. There are some universal guidelines to follow when purchasing an annuity for this purpose. The main requirements are that the annuity must be immediate, fixed, irrevocable, and non-transferable. Let us define those terms so we understand what they mean.

Fixed means the regular payment you receive from the annuity must always be the same.

You will receive only $1,200 per month for 20 years, for example. It will not be dependent on the up and down cycles of the stock market. It takes a number of years to be paid back for this investment.

Immediate means that you start to see the payments almost immediately after you purchase the annuity, which is the opposite of the deferred annuity. Irrevocable means you cannot change the terms or get your money back once you sign it and buy it. Non-transferable means that you cannot assign or transfer the ownership to anyone. You cannot sell it, and if you could, Medicaid would require you to use the money to pay your nursing home bill. So, it has no value as an asset because it cannot be sold. A single-premium immediate annuity is the only kind that Medicaid accepts. Some states are beginning to challenge this law and are trying to collect on the value by making it countable income.

The Deficit Reduction Act of 2005 makes any annuities purchased for Medicaid purposes as countable unless you name the state as one of the beneficiaries of the policy. This guarantees the state will not count the annuity you purchased as an asset.

Some disadvantages of Medicaid annuities are that they are a complex financial product and the amount you receive monthly may depend on the financial health of the insurance company you purchase the product from. Revocable annuities can incur large taxes if you withdraw money to use. For married couples, annuities can interfere with Medicaid rules protecting the community spouse. Annuities can decrease the amount of assets you are allowed to keep for couples applying for Medicaid. Some salespeople receive high commissions to sell these annuities, so a good lawyer should advise you on how to proceed with annuities. Annuities can be restrictive and some states may not allow them to be excluded. Many people who do not need them are buying annuities, unaware of the entire picture.

It is important for single or married persons purchasing Medicaid-friendly annuities to consult with an experienced elder lawyer, as these products are not always helpful for protecting assets.

Types of Annuities

An equity-fixed annuity allows individuals to participate in the stock market's ups and downs without losing the principal to unexpected market changes. It guarantees a minimum interest rate regardless of future performance. It is for active seniors who want to have the comfort of knowing the annuity is stable, but will get a larger return on their payment. It is a middle ground for those willing to take the risk to try something new.

A fixed annuity is a popular retirement and savings vehicle. It was created for long-term investors who want stability. It lets an insurance company invest your lump sum and gives you a higher return than on a CD product. It provides a tax-deferred benefit that lets you wait to pay taxes in the future. It takes place in two phases: the first is the long-term growth that happens on a tax-deferred basis; the second is where the annuity can be converted into a monthly fixed income and paid on a regular basis for a set number of years.

Fixed annuities can be purchased from insurance companies or financial institutions for a lump sum. Some annuities are paid periodically while the person is working. The money will earn a fixed rate of return. Often, you can negotiate the price of this product. The amount a product pays out varies, so it pays to shop around before purchasing one. There are two types of fixed annuities: life annuities and term-certain annuities.

With straight life annuities, the simplest form, the insurance component is based primarily on providing income until death. Once the payout period begins, the annuity pays a set amount per period to the person who owns it. It is less expensive than other types of annuities. They do not offer any money to beneficiaries after the annuitant's death. Those who want to leave something to family should purchase another type.

A sub-standard health annuity is a straight life annuity that someone with serious health problems can purchase. The annuities are priced with the consideration that the person may pass away. The lower the life expectancy, the more expensive the annuity is, because there is a reduced chance for the insurance company to make a return on the money the person invested. The person receives a lower percentage of his or her original investment. The payments are high because of the short-term life expectancy. Other insurance components are commonly not offered with this type of annuity.

Life annuities with a guaranteed term offer more of an insurance component. The person can name a beneficiary for the annuity. If the person passes away before term, the beneficiary will receive the sum of money not paid out. So in the event of an early death, they do not sacrifice their policy to the insurance agencies. This annuity comes at a high price.

Another aspect of life annuities with guaranteed terms is that beneficiaries receive one lump sum payment from the insurance company. This often results in an increase in the person's income, and they have to pay income tax on the sum they receive.

A joint life with last survivor annuity pays continued income to the spouse after the annuitant passes away. The payments are periodic rather than in one lump sum. The cost is higher for this type of annuity.

Term-certain annuities are a different product. They pay a given amount per period for a certain time no matter what happens to the person over the term. If the person dies before the term, the insurance company keeps the remainder of the value.

This type of annuity does not have an added insurance component. It does not account for health, life expectancy, or the beneficiaries. In the event of bad health or increased medical costs, the price of the annuity will not change to cover this; this type of annuity is less expensive because of this fact. The disadvantage of this kind of annuity is that once the term ends, so does the income from the annuity. This type of annuity is sold to those that want an inexpensive annuity to generate some income.

An immediate annuity lets you convert your savings income to an immediate stream of income for your needs. You will have the security of knowing you will receive money every month, even if you live until age 110. You can purchase this annuity using funds from your 401(k) or IRA, savings account, life insurance policy, or sale of your home. You get payment regularly either by check or automatic deposit into your checking account. You can choose how to receive payment — monthly, quarterly, or yearly. It is used to protect your assets from nursing home costs.

Immediate annuities are popular because seniors live much longer now. Annuities provide an immediate regular income for retirement that you will never outlive. They are a contract between you and the insurance company. Annuities are normally purchased with a large lump sum of money by conservative investors. Most are designed to pay expenses over a long period of time.

For example, a 75-year-old man buys a $100,000 annuity policy. Based on the interest rates and life expectancy, he will receive about $750 per month for the rest of his life. If he dies, his beneficiaries receive the remaining value. Immediate annuities offer a favorable tax treatment for older people. A large portion of the income is tax free.

Annuities are used for Medicaid planning purposes because when you purchase one, you remove the asset from your estate. This is not a good way to remove assets. You should consult an attorney before using this method.

A private annuity trust is an effective asset-management tool to handle sales of high-priced items, such as real estate, collectibles, stock, and other valuable assets. Many people get this trust to create a retirement plan, defer or eliminate real estate taxes, avoid probate, and protect family assets. It is a product used to create income for seniors. You transfer the asset you would like to sell into this trust and you are guaranteed a certain amount of payments for a certain period of time for life. The trust can then sell your real estate and use the money to invest in the trust that funds your regular lifetime income. It can protect assets for Medicaid planning.

Tips for Single Persons Purchasing Annuities for Medicaid

Some companies will not issue a policy for someone who is

over 85; other companies will go as high as 90. It is important to find out about the company before purchasing any product. Check with the Better Business Bureau or your local chamber of commerce for information. Most often, an annuity can be purchased for a single person in any amount. Another point to remember is that if the policy is based on life expectancy longer than the person purchasing the annuity, some part of the purchase price will be considered a gift to Medicaid.

It does not pay for a single person to buy an annuity in a state that requires it to be counted or used for Medicaid. Check with your state agency on rules before you purchase any annuity in your state for that particular purpose.

Most annuity contracts do not contain language or are not written to qualify for Medicaid rules. The monthly payment must be for life expectancy of the person purchasing the policy. The annuity cannot have any free look-back period in the contract and the value is agreed to all parties to be zero. The only value is the monthly income it generates. This feature as part of the contract is allowed in 29 states.

Commissions for Medicaid spend-down annuities are low while commissions on standard annuities are frequently higher. They sell you a product, but one that never qualifies for Medicaid. Always work with a qualified elder lawyer when you purchase a Medicaid annuity.

Many single persons over 65 are sold annuities that they are told are guaranteed not have to be counted by Medicaid. When the elderly person becomes ill and needs to go into the nursing home, they find the annuity is counted. They often have to sell or surrender the annuity and face heavy costs. They lose their assets because the annuity never protected their assets. So be careful when you buy a policy; make sure it will help you.

Most payments go to a nursing home or are used for allowable medical expenses. So for a Medicaid recipient, an annuity does not benefit the family in most cases.

If your parent is single and owns substantial retirement and savings accounts, it is not to the parent's benefit to buy an annuity. For those who have enough money to pay for their own care, they will get higher-quality long-term care than Medicaid provides. Whatever income your parent received from an annuity would almost certainly go to Medicaid. So, it may be wise not to purchase an annuity.

Do not forget about the Deficit Reduction Act 2005 that says if you purchase an annuity to protect your assets from Medicaid, the state must be named as one of the beneficiaries for them to not count the annuity. Always consult a good elder lawyer before purchasing an annuity.

Tips for Married Couples Purchasing Medicaid Annuities

A rule that recently changed is that any annuity purchased for Medicaid planning must name the state as a beneficiary. The state must be named the beneficiary after the community spouse and a disabled child, especially in cases of Medicaid patients receiving long-term care. The federal law changed the term from annuitant to institutionalized individual. When the community spouse purchases an annuity for a spouse in a nursing home, they must name the state beneficiary for the remaining payments after the person passes away. The spouse in the nursing home is known as the institutionalized individual.

If there is a surviving spouse or disabled child named as beneficiary of the annuity, the state will have to wait until the death of that person to collect on the debt. If the payments have stopped, there may be no funds available upon the death of the community spouse. It makes sense to purchase the shortest possible term annuity.

If the community spouse enters the nursing home after the nursing home spouse passes away, the state may request to be named beneficiary of the annuity or estate, so it gets the money for reimbursement of the Medicaid funding for the community spouse. The state will be repaid money only for the person who was put in a nursing home at the time the annuity was purchased.

In some states, the payment of the annuity to a community spouse can cause income of the spouse to exceed MMMNA. This will often be used by the nursing home as countable income.

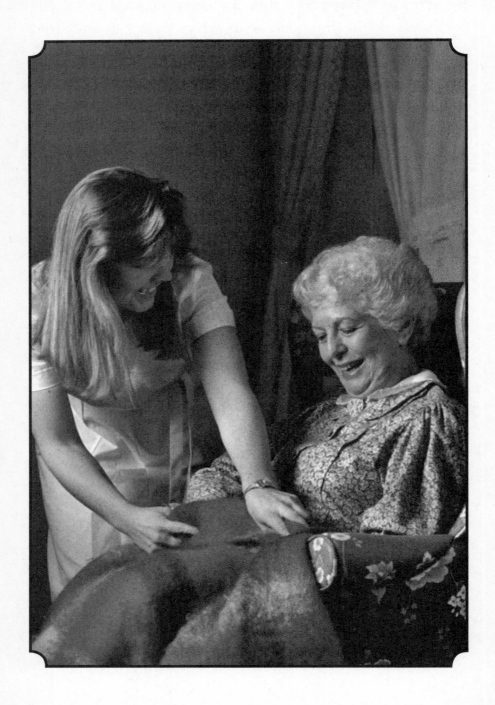

CHAPTER 6

Gifts

The rule states that if you make a gift to anyone other than your spouse, you are ineligible for Medicaid for a penalty period. Even if your income is within the range due to your penalty period, you will be denied coverage due to your gift.

A good time to apply is long before you run out or need the money. Owners of a home with equity over $500,000 will have to use some of the equity for Medicaid. Some suggest a reverse mortgage or home equity line. Do not transfer your home over to someone without thinking about it. First, you lose control over whether your home can be sold, mortgaged, or used for purposes you may not like. You might have problems with creditors, and an improper transfer may result in Medicaid denial should you apply for funds. Watch the value of your home. If the value exceeds a certain limit, that may disqualify you from Medicaid, unless you sell your home. Anyone loaning money for family business will be penalized, and if a loan is not repaid, that person may not be able to get Medicaid.

Medicaid Penalty Periods

Gifts to anyone but your spouse will make you ineligible to collect Medicaid for a certain period of time. The length of time this happens depends on the value of your gift and when it was made. Whether you are married or single, this law applies to you. There is no limit on the length of this penalty period.

As mentioned before, the look-back period has been increased from three years to five years. So, when giving away money or property to your family or friends, you may want to plan accordingly. The penalty period is determined by dividing the average cost of a nursing home in your state by the amount of the gift you made. Let us say you gave your son $60,000 on January 1, 2008. The average cost of the nursing home is $5,000 per month. Divide the $5,000 into the $60,000 to get an estimate of 12 months, or until January 1, 2009, for your penalty period.

The penalty period often begins when an individual applies for Medicaid and the assets are examined by the state. This new system discourages gift giving by anyone who may need long-term care in the next five years. The exceptions to these rules are: transfer to a spouse or third party for the benefit of the spouse; transfer to the disabled family member for the benefit of the disabled person; and transfer when imposing a penalty on the person or family would put a hardship on the family.

Any gifts given before February 8, 2006, are subject to a three-year look-back period. The new policy of a five-year look-back period with penalties has some of the following stipulations before it expires: the person is in a nursing home or has some Medicaid Waiver services; the person has applied for Medicaid; or the person is qualified for Medicaid.

Some states are working on Hardship Rules that will waive some of the penalty period and assets counted. States such as North Carolina have lobbied hard to get this into the rules for the state Medicaid applicants. There are many rules to interpret and fight for, but they will continue to work toward helping clients. Elder lawyers are often extremely helpful in getting clients waivers in Medicaid cases.

Value of the Gift

The value of a gift counted for Medicaid is determined by its fair market value at the time it is counted as an asset. The fair market value is the retail value or amount of money you would get by selling it to someone in the common public or for private sale.

For example, where do you find the value of an auto you may want to sell? Using the Kelley Blue Book or getting information from Consumer Reports can help you determine auto values; remember that one auto is excluded. For bank accounts, it is the cash value of the account when you liquidate it. With CDs, you only count the amount of interest credited to this account. The cash value of life insurance is counted so term life insurance has no value. Contact your insurance company for Form 712, which addresses this issue.

You can get an appraisal for real estate such as land and homes from a registered real estate agent. Sometimes, a recent tax bill may have the value of the entire property. Stock values fluctuate every day, so value must be taken on the day you received the gift.

Some people sell real estate or other items to their children for $1 or way below the retail value. This technique does not work, as it will be counted as a partial gift or sale. The amount received will be subtracted from the fair market value. In other words, if you sold your second car to your child for $2,000 when the car is truly worth $60,000, the $2,000 will be subtracted from the worth. Then, the $58,000 will be divided by the cost of nursing homes in your state.

Massachusetts has MassHealth, another name for Medicaid, which applies the five-year look-back period for gifts awfully strictly. For example, they monitor your checking and savings accounts for the last five years to see if any gifts were given. All withdrawals will be treated as gifts unless you are able to prove otherwise. A nursing home resident was found not eligible due to two gifts she made to her two sons worth $300. The attorney filed an appeal on this minor gift and the client was excused.

Look-Back Period

When you or your parent becomes ill, it is too late to transfer their home or money to qualify for Medicaid. If your father becomes ill, for example, and enters a nursing home, he cannot give his money away to your family. If both your parents are living, you can have the home transferred to the parent that is living in the house, and the state can only put a lien on your home in the worst-case scenario. It will be protected from estate recovery until the community spouse sells it or dies.

For example: Don adds his adult children to his deed on the house five years before applying for Medicaid. The house is worth $150,000. The adult children he adds to the deed are Tom and Alice. As long as Don keeps his name on the deed and resides in the house, his share is exempt from being counted by Medicaid. The portion of the house Don transferred to his children may not be exempt from being counted as an asset by Medicaid.

Anyone who wants to qualify for Medicaid should be planning in advance. If you give away assets even five years in advance just to qualify for Medicaid, you can face penalties and a period of being disqualified under the new laws. Consult a lawyer when planning for Medicaid and give away assets with the idea you will not need to utilize this service, as you will work at maintaining your health.

Irrevocable trusts are being used now with the new laws so people can remain in their homes. Maintaining and working hard at taking care of your physical and mental health is, of course, a sensible option. If clients need long-term care, the children can get money from a trust and sell the family home to raise money for nursing home care. If a person does not need long-term care until after five years, the person is protected and assets remain intact.

For those who need immediate care, a caregiver agreement is an option. This is when children are paid by their parents to help them, under the terms of a written agreement. The payments made to the children help to spend down the family assets so they can qualify for Medicaid. This child, who may have to take a leave from a job to care for the parent, is paid. This money is considered wages rather than a gift, so it avoids an asset transfer penalty. The family member must receive competitive wages and pay taxes on the money earned for caregiving services to their parents.

Gift Splitting

If you are married and a U. S. citizen, you can file an election on your gift-tax return that allows both you and your spouse to treat the gifts you made as equal. It gives credit equally to both of you for giving gifts, which is called gift splitting. For example, if you gave your sister $24,000 and your wife did not, you can elect that the $12,000 exclusion is covered by both of you; $12,000 was given by you, and $12,000 by your spouse. There will be no gift tax.

Another example is if you gave the Heart Association $12,000. If you split the gift between your spouse and yourself, the $6,000 is below the allowable limit, so you do not need to pay taxes on it. The Heart Association is a qualified charity, so you may get an income tax deduction for this gift. You need to file this when you make a gift that exceeds $12,000. These rules do not apply to Medicaid.

The 50/50 split transfer offers one way for a person to shorten the penalty period for gift giving or assets. The person gives half during the look-back period and keeps the other half. When the person seeks aid, the amount will be half of what it would have been if he or she gave away the entire amount. This technique applies to the look-back period of three years, but now it is five years.

Gift Trusts

Transferring money into a trust to benefit a grandchild with the help of an elder attorney is beneficial. You can specify when the principal and income will be available for the grandchild to use. You can even specify how the funds will be spent. Thus, you can reduce the size of your estate up to $12,000 in 2008. Although trusts own assets, you can still control them. Income earned by trusts that you deposit will not be taxed to you; trusts pay the taxes. They can be used for the benefit of your grandchildren and can be terminated when you choose.

Trusts may be suitable for those who have surplus capital and are sure they will never need regular withdrawals in the future. Individuals who feel confident they will live another seven years may benefit from the trusts. The amount that is invested is put into a life insurance investment bond that is gifted to a Discounted Gift Trust; it will be exempt for gift tax purposes. The owner will be entitled to regular withdrawals determined when the trust is created; it provides lifetime income. Often, payments cease when the owner dies.

Long-Term Life Insurance and Gifts

Under new Medicaid laws, the government is encouraging those over 65 to take more responsibility should they need long-term healthcare. Many individuals are encouraged to purchase long-term health insurance to cover costs of nursing home and healthcare. Many seniors will not purchase policies because they are too expensive and risky.

With new laws, those who purchase long-term care insurance during the five-year look-back period will find these policies do not cover the cost of the care they need. In states such as New York and Connecticut, nursing home costs can sometimes exceed $10,000 per month, while most average citizens cannot even afford policies that run between $3,000 and $6,000 per year.

Some states are working to address this problem by finding exceptions to the Medicaid rules. Others are working with insurance providers to try to develop a long-term health insurance plan that helps consumers and the healthcare industry.

The healthcare industry is offering plans with a shorter benefit period. This cuts the price of the monthly or yearly premium. If you do not think you will develop a long-term illness, it may be pointless to buy a policy with long-term benefits. Married couples may be better off buying a shared policy instead of two separate ones. It is cheaper than buying two policies with lifetime benefits. Often, both spouses do not need care at the same time, so this saves money. A family history of long-term illnesses might warrant purchase of a policy. The younger you are, the lower the premiums. For example, if you are in your 50s, premiums will be lower if you purchase now than they would be if you wait until you are in your 60s.

The possibility of needing a long-term care policy should be considered by anyone over 65. This policy helps pay for services that may not be covered and are exceedingly expensive. These policies can give you control over long-term care services you receive and where you will receive them. It can assist with help in your home with bathing, dressing, eating, and cleaning. Some policies cover community-care programs like adult daycare and assisted living services that are provided in special settings other than your home. Other policies cover visiting nurses and nursing home services.

If you wait until you are 70 or 80, the cost of the policy will be astronomical. Some have restrictions on age and health. The average cost of a policy of someone 65 or older in good health ranges from $2,000 to $3,000 per year. Do not purchase a policy if you cannot afford what you need or have to lower your standard of living. Some points to consider when purchasing a policy are:

- **Coverage is important.** Some policies only cover nursing home care or in-home care. Some include nursing homes, assisted living centers and adult daycare. Look for what you need for yourself. Some even pay for family or friends to care for you in your own home.

- **Benefit periods ranges from two to six years or the rest of your life.** If the policy has an elimination or waiting period, you pay out of pocket expenses for 0 to 100 days, which lowers the monthly premium considerably. The policy should have inflation protection included. It should not require you to spend time in the hospital before benefits begin. The policy should be renewed as long as you pay the premiums. It should have one deductible and allow you to downgrade coverage if you cannot afford the premiums. It should include coverage for dementia.

Do not purchase a policy if you cannot afford the premiums

or it lacks a home care coverage clause. If you do not want to go into a nursing home at all, consider other ways to deal with the problem. The return rate for policies is 60 to 65 percent.

Gift Taxes

The gift-tax exclusion of $12,000 per person is not the same as the Medicaid exclusion for gifts. Under federal rules, any gift made to another person over $12,000 means you do not need to file a gift-tax exclusion, if your gifts do not exceed $12,000 per year.

There are no exclusions for figuring a Medicaid gift. If you give away $50,000 to one or five people, it will be counted the same. They will tally up the amount of gifts within the last five years and add the total. Then, they will divide the average cost of a nursing home in your state to determine when you will be eligible. Exceptions are gifts to a spouse or a trust for a disabled child. If you give a gift to someone for $12,000, it will be counted as an asset for Medicaid eligibility.

Purchasing a policy for five or more years is a smart idea, with the look-back period now up to five years. After that, you can give away assets and apply for Medicaid five years from the date you made the gift. Your insurance policy will be in place in the event that you do not get Medicaid. Determining your gift is easier when you have long-term health insurance in place. So, wait until your long-term policy is in place before you start transferring assets.

Cons of Long-Term Health Insurance

A Consumer Reports study of 47 insurance policies revealed that long-term health insurance is too expensive and does not cover enough to make it worth paying for. So, most elderly persons should not rush out to purchase it. The good news is that it is improving and companies are offering more options in this area. The policies are becoming better and less expensive.

Conversely, with long-term care insurance being so expensive and Medicaid harder to qualify for, it is well worth looking into as an option for the future. If you are well-off financially, it may well be worth purchasing a policy for yourself or an elderly family member. The problems with the policies are that some companies may not stay in business or cover what you believe they will when the time comes to collect the benefits. Look carefully at policies and make sure they specify what they cover and the terms in clear understandable language.

Generation-Skipping Transfer Tax

This tax is confusing but the premise is that it is a tax separate from income, and estate and gift taxes. It is supposed to trap the transfer of property between successive generations. In other words, it allows transfers of property to spouses and children with taxes going to the grandchildren or those deemed to be two generations below the person making the transfers. It is a steep tax — about 55 percent of the value of the property. It drops from 55 percent to 45 percent from 2007 through 2010. Those who transfer all of their property to the next generation do not have to worry about this tax. No tax is imposed on this level. Every individual is allowed $1.5 million generation skipping exemption since 2004. Many get around this tax by only transferring property to next generation such as parents to sons and daughters. For more information on how this tax may apply to you, consult a qualified financial planner or consultant.

This tax usually applies to grandchildren or great grand-children who received a transfer of money or trust from family member. The person must be 37 ½ years younger than the person who gave the gift or trust. The recipient must pay tax on the distribution.

CHAPTER 7

Wills and Deeds

It is often not enough to have a will to protect your assets from Medicaid — now you need more. There are different types of wills that can be prepared by an attorney. A will is a legal document that tells how a person's property should be handled when they die. A will should be written to express the wishes of the person requesting it. Married couples can prepare wills that address inheritance-tax protection and the issue of long-term healthcare. By making arrangements, you can ensure your spouse will have quality arrangements and medical care.

A well spouse can take action and make sure that if something happened to them, all assets can pass into a special needs trust for the ill spouse. All assets will be protected; then the person can apply for Medicaid. A holographic will is one written without witnesses, but few states recognize these wills as legal. Oral wills are also recognized in few states and only in compelling situations like impending death. A self-proving will is one that has been witnessed and signed. It has been created with all the formalities required by state law. It can have an attached affidavit signed by a notary public.

A formal will is used in probate. It is put in writing and signed by the person making the will and another witness.

What Should Be in a Will?

A will should state that you are of sound mind at the time when you sign it. The names, birth dates, and locations of all children, relatives, and friends in the will should be stated clearly. You should talk with a lawyer about whether to name stepchildren or illegitimate children in the will. You would do this to avoid claims that might come up if you leave them out after your die, or even before.

Appointment of a guardian for any children or stepchildren should be addressed. Consult your lawyer to discuss whether you should have a separate lawyer for your finances. A detailed list of who will inherit specific items of property is often included. Some states keep separate lists with the will, so it can be updated periodically.

The division of property should be fair. Sometimes, making provisions through a testamentary trust for minors and those who tend to waste money is a good idea. When heirs have the same name, they must be clearly identified with numbers to tell the difference between them.

Do not put your organ donor wishes in your will or funeral arrangements; most wills are read after the funeral. Only describe the assets you wish to leave to your heirs, but not all of them. It is advisable to try to avoid inflexible instructions like selling all assets —leave that to your executor and heirs. Finally, avoid ambiguous wording as much as possible.

Burial instructions are often included in a will. It is a good idea to have them written up in a separate statement that can be accessed. You may want to have a copy of the will in a separate place specifically for burial instructions.

The will should be kept in a safe place like a safe-deposit box. You will have to arrange for an executor to have access to the box after your death. Some states put a freeze on the box when you die.

Different Types of Wills

Oral wills are spoken to a witness instead of being written down. They are often used by those who feel there is not enough time to draft a document. Frequently, armed service members in active combat make an oral will; fellow soldiers serve as witnesses for the will. This is one type of oral will that most probate courts will recognize. This type of will is not normally recommended due to the possibility of fraud and misinterpretation.

A deathbed will is drafted when someone is facing imminent death. They are often hard to prove legally and are often challenged by family members. Although the person is obviously not sound of body, the person still can be of sound mind when facing death. These wills are supposed to be witnessed by two or more people.

Holographic wills are informal and handwritten. Not all states will recognize this sort of will. They must be signed by the person making the will and another witness. They are frequently used when something unexpected or tragic happens. A probate court often finds them invalid.

Self-probating wills are considered time savers. When the will is created, a witness signs a statement that the person creating the will was of sound mind. These documents are important because without them, the witness would have to testify in probate court. These wills are created with an attorney and are the least likely to be challenged in court.

Changing or Challenging a Will

Revising a will is often necessary when you divorce, if you marry, become a widow or widower, have a child or adopt one. When a beneficiary or someone in your will dies, you will want to change it. If you want to change how your property will be distributed, you have to rewrite the will. When you move into another state, your net worth increases dramatically.

A will can be revised, and this is called a codicil or a formal amendment to the will. Preparing a new will or revoking a prior will is sometimes necessary due to changing circumstances in your life.

A professional should always make the changes. Sometimes, a person wants to change how his or her assets are divided or remove a person who has fallen out of favor or who has died. Sometimes, a person may want to give money to a charity or favorite cause.

Only persons of legal standing can contest wills— a spouse or child, for example, who should have been included in the will but was not. Wills can be challenged for fairness. Some of the reasons a will is challenged are that the document is suspected to be a forgery, the person was not of sound mind when the will was drafted, or the will did not meet the requirements of the state.

Disinheriting a person is more common in wills than people think. To keep children or grandchildren from receiving assets from your estate, you must legally disinherit them by saying so in your will. Spouses are harder to disinherit. Most attorneys will discourage their client from disinheriting someone in a will.

Divorce can sometimes complicate a will. In some states, divorce makes a will invalid. In others, the parts that refer to the spouse are revoked.

Dying without a will is known as dying intestate, which is a common occurrence. In all cases, probate appoints a personal representative to be in charge of the assets. The administrator pays all debts and the rest is divided among beneficiaries.

Lady Bird Deeds or Enhanced Life Estate Deeds

Most families own property that they want to give or pass on to family members. One way is to add their names to the deed on your house and land. This method can be full of problems and red tape.

Another way is make a Lady Bird deed, which is also known as the transfer on death deed. It works when the owners or grantors deed the property to the children. They reserve a life estate for themselves with the option to sell the property at any time if needed. The deed means the grantors still own the property. The grantor can sell the property at any time. If the grantor never sells the property, it goes to the grantees.

The Lady Bird deed has many virtues. It bypasses probate for real property. It does not result in capital gains and is valued on what it is worth on the day of the last grantor's death, which is called stepped-up value.

It does not open up the property to creditors because grantees do not have much interest until the grantor has passes away and only if the home was never sold. It allows the grantor to sell the property at any time if needed for medical purposes.

The deed is named after Lady Bird Johnson, the First Lady of the United States from 1963 to 1969, who inherited property from her husband, Lyndon B. Johnson, from one of these deeds. It is not used that much because trusts are more expensive then wills and more complicated to set up. This deed avoids a costly probate process. The states of California, Texas, Ohio, Florida and many others now use this deed.

The deed is also called an enhanced life estate deed, a mechanism to bypass the probate process. The husband and wife retain the right to live in the property for life. They control what happens to the property so at any time, they can sell or revoke the deed. Individuals or couples who want to simplify the transfer of their property upon death while retaining full control of it while alive can use it. Medicaid eligibility will not be affected, as long as the intent to return to the home is demonstrated. This deed is good for a woman who wants to pass on the property to her children without probate, but wishes to remain in control of her estate.

Do not put your children's names as joint tenants with rights of survivorship. If you do this, the property may not be protected from creditors, so in effect, you can lose your lifetime protection. You might be disqualified from Medicaid should you have to go a nursing home. You may have to pay a heavy gift tax and you may not be able to sell your home if you choose to. A person can sell or change the deed without notifying the beneficiaries.

Sometimes, a quitclaim deed is made to make it easier for the family. The problem with this is that the owner would not be able to mortgage or sell the property without the consent of the beneficiaries. It is often used to avoid probate.

Beneficiary Deeds

A beneficiary deed will disqualify a person who needs long-term care from receiving Medicaid benefits. When it comes to real estate, this deed does not allow the person to name a beneficiary in most states. Transferring property requires a probate hearing along with the expense.

Transferring real estate at death is easier now in Colorado by means of what it is called a beneficiary deed. It is made by the property owner and recorded in real estate records. The deed can be revoked at any time before the death of the owner.

There are many issues to consider before making such a simple deed. Anyone who thinks they will apply for Medicaid should not make this type of deed. It will disqualify the person from Medicaid as long as the deed is in effect. If a parent leaves the property to three children and one child dies, the two left will inherit the property. It does not sever joint tenancy. It cannot be used to avoid the debts of the deceased.

Cheaper than a living trust, a beneficiary deed has no gift-tax liability. It can be changed at any time or revoked. Since the property is not transferred until the death of the last owner, its value remains in the estate of the deceased for estate tax purposes. When there are several beneficiaries, they each own interest in the property. It can make the property hard to manage or control.

Joint Owners with Rights of Survivorship

The most common method of avoiding probate and passing on property after your death is joint ownership with rights of survivorship. There are two common forms of joint ownership. One is called tenancy by the entirety. If husband and wife own the property, neither can dispose or sell the property without the consent of the other. When one spouse dies, the entire property passes to the other spouse. Creditors who have a judgment against one spouse cannot collect a judgment by seizing property.

The other form of joint ownership allows for survivorship rights between or among two or more people, who are not necessarily husband and wife. The result is that the last surviving joint owner receives full ownership. The difference is that any of the parties can give away their share by selling or giving away their interests. Common forms of property this relates to are autos, bank accounts, and real estate.

Advantages of joint ownership are that property passes to the surviving co-owners automatically. Often, only a death certificate is needed to deal with the property. Joint bank accounts offer a married couple convenience and flexibility. Funds are immediately available if one spouse dies or is incapacitated. These arrangements are suitable to married couples, especially if someone wants to remain living in the house.

One of the disadvantages of joint ownership is loss of control over property. Another is a problem getting rid of the property or obtaining loans. Serious legal problems and an increase in the cost of probate can occur. Cumbersome conservatorship proceedings and disagreements between owners that may cost in terms of time and money are also negatives of this type of ownership.

Joint tenancy is a way to own property together. Each state has their own rules by incorporating the following guidelines:

- Both parties must receive ownership rights at the same time.

- A unity of title means both persons are on the same deed or document as owners.

- Both tenants must own equal shares of the property ,and both tenants have rights to occupy, enjoy, and use the property.

Executors and Trustees

One of the most important decisions you will make is to pick the person in charge of your assets. What is an executor? An executor is someone you select to carry out your arrangements after death. This can include your funeral arrangements, paying your debts, arranging for the distribution of your assets and representing your affairs. An executor will collect the assets of the estate, protect the estate property, prepare an inventory of the property, pay valid claims against the estate, represent the estate in claims against others, and distribute the estate property to beneficiaries.

One option is to appoint a paid executor with no conflicts of interest. This is why some families often do not name family members or business partners. If you have several beneficiaries who do not get along, you may want an outside beneficiary. The larger the estate, the more potential for conflict; as a result, it may be wise to name an outside executor. There are several good reasons to choose someone other than your spouse. He or she may be grief stricken or have a serious disability. If you think your spouse may not be up to the job, consider a lawyer.

Most people opt for unpaid executors because of the steep fees that a lawyer charges. Many people choose a friend or family member. What should you look for in an executor? A person who is capable of the job would be someone who is persistent and detail-oriented, and who can deal with medical bills and issues. It should be someone who has the time and patience to deal with paperwork and relatives who may inquire about money.

What Is a Trustee?

If you leave money in a trust, the trustee is the person responsible for distributing and dealing with the details of the trust to your beneficiaries. Trustees may need to collect estate taxes, invest money, pay bills, file accounting, and pay beneficiaries. A person who can deal with your beneficiaries easily, such as a bank or trust company, should be appointed as a backup. It is hard to decide whether to use a professional or family member.

There are pros and cons of appointing a family member. It can be good if the person has time and wants to do the job. Family members may not mind family conflicts and want to see the trust work effectively.

Drawbacks are that your family member may lack expertise to do the job. Trustees can be long-term, but relatives, die banks or trust companies are frequently not. Family members can fight, making it hard to carry out the terms of trust for trustee.

Choosing an institutional trustee has pros and cons too. You can expect to pay for these services. It can be costly for a small trust. Banks are impersonal and may not take an individual interest in your trust or how it does. So you may want to talk to other members involved in the trust to see what they think.

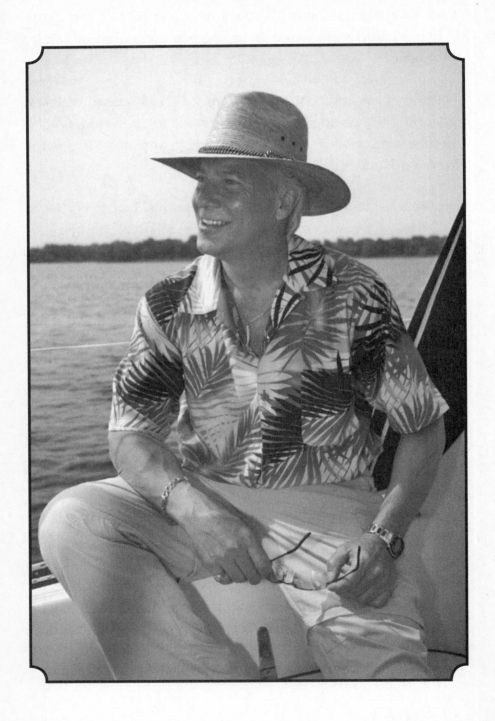

CHAPTER 8

Creative Ways to Qualify for Medicaid

Do not try to hide your income to qualify for Medicaid. When you apply for Medicaid, not mentioning your assets or gifts you made is illegal and reason to be disqualified from ever receiving assistance. Medicaid fraud carries some severe penalties and there are several different kinds. Let us review some.

Those who receive Medicaid commit fraud by loaning their Medicaid identification card to another person. Some forge medical prescriptions for drugs. Some use multiple Medicaid ID cards. Some receive duplicate or excessive services for the same health services, or resell items provided by Medicaid.

Some providers engage in fraud that delivers the services of healthcare facilities and doctors, for example. They can be dentists, doctors, clinics, nursing home, or personal assistants who cheat the system. Examples would be: a home attendant billing her grandmother about $20,000 for services she never provided, and Medicaid paid her; a doctor billing for tests never performed; billing private insurance *and* Medicaid, getting paid twice; requiring the patient to return for another appointment when it is not necessary; unnecessary X-rays and blood work; billing for extra services or for two offices when the patient went to one; billing for additional people in the family who never went to the doctor's office or clinic. One dentist billed Medicaid thousands of dollars for services she never performed. She was not monitored until a few years later, then she was arrested and convicted of fraud.

Another case of fraud occurred when an overweight woman received a prescription drug for AIDS, which she claimed to have. The drug, a synthetic hormone called Serotism, cost $6,400 a month. The woman sold the drug to bodybuilders as a steroid to bulk up. The woman also stole another person's card, which is another form of Medicaid fraud. In New York, physicians under Medicaid wrote many prescriptions for this drug, which was being used illegally for bodybuilders and athletes who wanted to improve muscle mass.

Other common fraud scenarios are: a physician billing Medicaid for doctor visits when vacationing, a nurse submitting false time sheets for patients who were never there, and a clinic billing for therapy sessions that never took place.

A pharmaceutical company overpriced a prescription drug, thus collecting more money than the drug was worth. The penalty for this crime was that the company had to pay back $1.4 million dollars for three prescription drugs they overcharged consumers for. They were supposed to report prices accurately, but inflated them to make money. Two of the drugs prevent vomiting and the other was an antibiotic.

Another company in Missouri billed Medicaid for home dialysis services, but overcharged for the services and collected more than allowed. They billed for tests not needed and paid kickbacks to physicians. They were fined heavily for fraud. Dialysis removes toxins from the blood when a patient's kidneys cannot do it. Some forms of dialysis can be done at home.

Other cases of Medicaid fraud include a dentist who claimed to see 991 patients a day, and a school district assigning dozens of students to Medicaid speech therapy.

Damages for Medicaid fraud are liable to the federal government for payment from two to three times the amount of benefits received wrongfully. You can pay from $5,000 to $10,000 for each false medical claim file. You can receive a criminal penalty up to one year in prison and a $10,000 fine and not be eligible to receive Medicaid for one year. Anyone who files a lawsuit against you for the government is rewarded 15 to 30 percent of the penalties. In some cases, you will never be able to receive Medicaid again under any circumstances.

Tips on Medicaid Spend Down

Spend Down is the process of reducing your assets to qualify for Medicaid. It is, in essence, spending your money until the asset limit is met. The asset limit in the state of New Jersey is $2,000 for the Medicaid Only program and $4,000 for the Medically Needy program. A person must be 65 years or older and have limited income to qualify.

Some people have too much income to qualify for Medicaid when they need it for long-term medical care; this is called excess income. Some people can qualify if their medical bills are equal to or greater than the excess. The classic way to spend down is to pay nursing home bills with your own money until your reduced savings lets you qualify. Another way is to convert countable assets to non-countable ones by spending money on something that will benefit you and the family. To be eligible for spend down, you must be disabled, blind, or at least 65 years or older, and need long-term nursing care.

Home improvements can help you with spend down, as your home is excluded from being counted as an asset. Since you can leave your house to your family members, any money you use for home improvements is wise. Repair your roof, remodel that outdated kitchen, pave that driveway, put in a new furnace, rewire the electrical system for safety, and build an addition for your mother-in-law. These projects will cost thousands and reduce your Medicaid countable assets. Do you need new appliances? How about new windows and doors to make your home energy efficient? Do you need a new heating system or central air conditioning? Have you thought of trying solar energy? Anything that adds to your home's value is a way to spend your money wisely.

Do you dream of a bigger home? Sell your older, smaller house and move into a newer one. This is another way to spend down your money. Remember, the equity in your home cannot exceed $500,000. Now you can qualify for tax sheltering every two years. All personal property is excluded, so you can buy clothes, shoes, towels, and appliances, just to name a few. Do you dream of having a subzero built-in refrigerator or a space-age kitchen stove? Do not get carried away with this before you qualify for Medicaid, or you may have to pay it back or have it counted. An auto is excluded, so why not get a bigger, more expensive one if you can afford it? A newer or larger car with more features is a good way to move that countable income to non-countable column. Do not buy a sports car, but something that is practical and will help you in the long run; perhaps a van for a larger family or something where you can store your bike for those long trips to the country.

If you prepay for funeral and burial expenses, this will not be included or counted. Paying out your own expenses gives you peace of mind and spares your family more grief when the time comes to deal with your or their deaths. The average cost of a funeral or burial is $8,500 to $10,000. Paying costs ahead of time is a good way to spend down your excess funds.

Purchase long-term health insurance for nursing home costs. This can be an extremely useful way to spend income, as this insurance is extremely expensive to begin with. You can purchase long-term health insurance even if you are in a nursing home.

Get all your dental work done, as Medicaid does not cover dental work that well. Get those dentures made or bridge work done and pay up front. Dental work is expensive and it pays to have your work done. If you need a hearing aid, get one now, as they are expensive and make a big difference in your hearing. Check your eyes and invest in good glasses or contacts.

Buy anything that will make your life more comfortable in the long run: a new living room set, or a new mattress for your bad back. Pay to get your house as comfortable as possible for you to live there in your golden years; this is a practical and easy way to spend down your money. Get those needed railings in your bathroom or other rooms. Do you need a ramp or special entrance way? Make your home as easy to maintain as possible. Fix what you have to, so you are not struggling with repairs later.

Long-Term Care Insurance

Long-term care insurance is a relatively new type of health insurance that covers long-term illness and nursing home costs. With the problems of Medicaid, it is being pushed as an alternative to depending on qualifying for Medicaid. It is actually administered more often through adult daycare centers, assisted living centers, home health agencies, and retirement communities. It covers expenses for medical bills from long-term care for the elderly or disabled. This insurance might prevent your family from financial ruin. It also might cover services that help you stay in your home longer. Long-term care is expensive and may not be needed if situations change. There are two types of policies: facility and comprehensive. Facility covers only nursing home care, while comprehensive covers both home care and nursing homes. Comprehensive is more expensive.

What is the right time to buy a policy? Some say when you are in your 50s or 60s. It can cost between $2,000 to $3,000 per year. Often, the policy covers nursing home care. Be sure you can afford the premiums before you decide to buy a policy.

Consider whether the policy pays for just nursing home care or care for services at your home while you are still living independently. Some policies cover a mixture of care options, so shop wisely. Some even will pay a family member or friend to care for you at home. You can purchase a policy from two to six years. There may be a waiting period with out-of-pocket expenses in which you must wait for on average 100 days before coverage begins; you will need to pay your bills until then. A non-forfeiture will continue to pay for your care even if you stop making payments.

Some important questions to consider are the following:

- Will you receive benefits without hospitalization?

- Will the policy be renewed as long as you pay the premiums?

- Does it have one deductible for the life of the policy?

- Does it avoid pre-existing conditions should you disclose them?

- Does it offer inflation protection and allow you to lower your premium payment if you need to?

- Does it include coverage for dementia?

- Does it include at least one year nursing care and home healthcare?

- Does it allow you to cancel the policy after 30 days if you choose?

When reviewing policies, look at the daily benefit, the amount you receive from the insurance company for your daily care. You can, on average, select $400 to $500 daily. Find out what the current daily rate in your state is. What is the benefit period? Two or three years is an average policy because that is the length of a typical nursing home stay. It can range from $3,600 to $10,000 per year for a good policy.

The cons include some especially high premiums that you may not be able to afford. You may never need the services or federal insurance may pay for your care. You may qualify for Medicaid if your assets are low. Other options such as a reverse mortgage or trust might work better than this. Long-term insurance may be limited despite the high cost.

What is the difference between a tax-qualified policy and a non-tax qualified policy? A tax-qualified policy may offer a tax deduction on your policy or premiums. To qualify for the tax break, you must be certified by a health professional as having a chronic illness for at least 90 days. You must be unable to perform two out of five activities of daily living. Cognitive impairment must be severe and require extensive supervision. If you claim this deduction, you must itemize your medical expenses. They are subject to age-related limits.

A non-tax qualified policy for benefits received after January 1, 1997, will not be taxed and does not require certification over 90 days to access benefits. Those who have care for less than 90 days still get benefit payments. They do not have the limits of daily living activities restriction. No portion of the premium is deductible.

Irrevocable Life Insurance

If your home equity is above the state limit, you have to reduce it to qualify for Medicaid. How do you do this?

A reverse mortgage is a loan against your house that you do not have to pay back as long as you live there. It helps you turn your home value into cash without moving or repaying the mortgage each month. It can be paid to you in a single lump sum, monthly cash advance, or a credit line that lets you decide when and how much of the available cash is paid to you. No matter how this loan is paid out to you, you do not have to pay it back until you die, move out, or sell your home. To be eligible for most reverse mortgages, you must be 62 years or older and own your own home. This allows you to stay in your home and upgrade it, using the money you get from this loan; many seniors are opting to do this. Reverse mortgages help with home improvements, income supplementation, and medical expenses.

Reverse mortgages may not always be the best idea. If no one lives in the house and you are in a nursing home, you would not get a reverse mortgage. If an owner takes a reverse mortgage and has to go into a nursing home, the mortgage will be paid off within one year of the owner moving out. This often forces a sale of the house, thus making it countable income to the nursing home.

Obtain a home equity loan. How would an ill person in a nursing home pay back the loan? Once on Medicaid, you cannot use money to pay the loan. This works only if family members are willing to keep paying the home equity loan. Perhaps, family members can pay the loan in exchange for ownership or shares in the house.

You can deed the whole or part of the house to a family member. Another option is to transfer a small percentage to one or more children. The homeowner borrows money from family members in exchange for interest in the house or part ownership.

IRAs are countable assets for Medicaid. You can transfer your IRA to a retirement annuity, making the IRA not countable. This is one idea if you need to convert it to an asset that is not counted.

Income-producing property is excluded. Medicaid will count the income generated but not the property itself. "Property" can mean real estate and other items such as jewelry, furniture, and autos, as opposed to bank accounts.

Spousal Refusal

A U. S. district court upheld the right of a nursing home spouse to expect support from the state and have their spouse refuse to support them. Mrs. Clara Morenz filed a document with the state, refusing to provide her husband with financial assistance for nursing home costs. She had transferred a large part of the money into her name. The state cannot consider the income or assets of the community spouse. If you have the money, a lawsuit in your state may save you money that would be wasted on long-term medical care. Legally, you are not responsible for the care of your spouse or elderly parents. Spousal refusal may work for regular working couples with average assets that do not exceed limits.

Mr. Morenz applied for Medicaid in January 2004 after living in a nursing home since 2000. His wife lived in the family homestead. His wife filed a legal document with the state of Connecticut refusing to pay any of his nursing home costs. In the 36 months before applying for Medicaid, he had transferred his $323,131 in assets to Mrs. Morenz using a durable power of attorney. He was refused Medicaid, but later the federal court moved that she could keep the money and the state had to pay his medical bills. He also transferred assets in the look-back period of 36 months, which now has changed to 60 months or five years.

Medicaid views spousal refusal as a way for people to keep wealth and force Medicaid to foot the bill. States can challenge spousal refusal if the state believes the law was violated. In New York, Medicaid lawyers have won more than $2.5 million in recovered assets in lawsuits against more affluent people. They do not want to see the wealthy on Medicaid.

Many states may change the spousal refusal law because they do not want similar cases being tried in their state. They will look at the language of this clause if they have it, though not all states support this clause. Still, the state of Connecticut can still try to claim estate recovery after Mrs. Morenz passes away for costs covered by Medicaid of her husband for nursing home care.

Children as Paid Caregivers

It comes as a shock to some families that adult children are not legally obligated to care for their elderly parents. Parents can reduce countable assets by paying their children for non-medical care services. A child can contract with the parent to provide personal care such as transportation, meals, housekeeping, and lawn care just like commercial companies.

A contract should follow a few of the following guidelines:

- Prepare a detailed written contract for delivery of services including hourly rate and time spent.

- Both parents and the person in the family doing the service should sign the agreement.

- The signature should be dated and notarized at the time of signing.

- The rates charged should be comparable to other commercial ventures.

- Find out what other professional agencies charge in your area by calling up a few agencies and getting estimates.

- Keep good records. This is a good way to spend money to get assets reduced for Medicaid.

The adult child who is working for the parent should check with his or her accountant about reporting the contract. Is this is an employee or independent contractor situation? Find out more about income tax withholding, Social Security, Medicare, and reporting to the IRS below.

Sometimes, when a child finds out they can charge for taking care of their parents, they say, "I have been taking care of Dad for four years. Can I get paid." The truth is that you cannot get paid unless you had a written contract in place. So this retroactive argument does not hold any credibility. Medicaid will say you did it out of moral obligation or love, so there is no reimbursement.

In Arizona, for example, a spouse can be paid for basic care of that person's husband or wife in a long-term care system. A woman caring for her sick husband who gets a disability payment finds being paid for her care of him incredibly helpful financially. Medicaid pays for meal preparation, bathing, and household chores. The caregivers must go through formal training and the person cared for must agree to it. Caregivers receive about $10 per hour.

Sometimes, family caregiving is not beneficial. According to police reports, an 84-year-old farmer deeded his house to his daughter, son-in-law, and kids. When he complained he was not receiving proper attention, his family became verbally abusive and his son-in-law hit him in the face. The conflict escalated and the elderly man had to get a restraining order against the daughter's husband, who had moved into a trailer on the property. The daughter also shoved her father into a fence and to the ground. Such situations where elder abuse takes place must be checked on and supervised. Caregiving is tremendously stressful and often, not all families foster caring relationships. It is important to check on and monitor the elderly being cared for at home by family members, especially when state funds are being used.

Cash and Counseling is a program designed to meet serious problems that Medicaid patients have getting personal assistance in a home for illness. It covers simple services such as bathing, dressing, grooming, and meal preparation. It allows ill people to hire home health aides and have control over services, which gives seniors more independence. Some senior use their own children, since it is a supervised program and is more successful than non-supervised situations. For instance, Brenda Terry gives paid care to her mother, who needs help after a stroke. She is able to stay home with her and be paid by the Cash and Counseling program. Her mother's health has improved considerably.

Louis lives near his parent's house in a separate apartment. He has received personal assistance since 1990 through a

Medicaid waiver program. This allows him to hire his own worker. He has a close family friend of 12 years help him with everything from dressing, undressing, toileting, cooking, and transportation. In June 2006, he switched from the waiver program to a Cash and Counseling program called Personal Choices. This program allows him to pay his longtime worker more per hour than he could before. He is excited about the added flexibility in the budget. He can pay his friend and save money for other things.

Calvin, who is blind, was struck by a car and has impaired coordination. He also needs dialysis for kidney disease three times a week. He has participated in a program called New Jersey Cash and Carry Personal Preference, which has helped alleviate some of his frustration with the programs he used. His sister helps him twice a day and he has ordered a voice-activated microwave, with which he can prepare his own meals, and computer equipment allowing him to order food online. The program gives him more control and independence.

Overall, patients with the Cash and Counseling program are more satisfied with their care. They receive help with housekeeping, meals, and other household chores. The program relieves the burdens of family caregivers and helps patients with a feeling of independence. It gives consumers flexibility without costing Medicaid more.

Contracts for paid family caregiving should be made with an attorney so that they meet legal and tax regulations. A contract for services may not disqualify you from qualifying for Medicaid. It is important to discuss the contract with relatives or siblings to avoid family disagreements.

It is sometimes hard for elderly patients to pay their family members when it is normally something one does for free. Some elderly patients may not want to pay relatives or feel resentful because they have to do so.

A contract should pay the fair market price for services. It should specify how the payment will be rendered in weekly, monthly, or one lump sum based on the life expectancy of the senior. Some contracts deposit money into an escrow account instead of giving it directly to the person.

Warnings on Limited Family Partnerships

A limited family partnership is a legal partnership in which only family members are partners. An example is parents and children all investing in owning a house. An agreement is drawn up, giving each person a certain percentage of ownership. This is not a good tool for Medicaid because many states say this is a technique of giving gifts to family members, so it will be counted and not ignored.

The partnership becomes its own entity and has its own tax identification number. It can conduct the same activities as a corporation or individual. One advantage is that partners cannot distribute or sell the interest, keeping the wealth in the family. All members of the partnership must agree upon any changes made. Major conflicts can be settled through arbitration.

The valuation discount is a big plus. A gift at 10 percent in a $1,000,000 limited partnership has lower value than a regular gift given to someone without this partnership. The tax paid would be significantly reduced.

This partnership is useful in reducing gift and estate taxes, allowing parents to shift wealth to their children. Sometimes, children can manage assets for the parents, though they receive most of the income. Upon the parent's death, the assets are distributed without going through probate. The partners cannot make investment decisions, force a partner to buy an interest, or dissolve the partnership. The parents give up assets, but still have control. Sometimes, the parents own 1 percent and the children own the rest.

A partnership reduces the value of the estate through use of valuation discounts. This means the principal sum of family limited partnership interest is less than the value of underlying assets held by the partnership. This is due to the lack of control and marketability of ownership units. Medicaid may not count as the partnership.

Non-tax advantages include:

- Preserving liquid assets by giving children a non-spendable limited partnership rather than securities or cash.

- The children are protected from claims of a divorcing spouse; control remains with the family unit.

- The agreement can be amended at any time.

- You achieve significant gift-tax discounts due to lack of marketability.

- Control of the partnership and income can be split among family members based on the percentage of ownership.

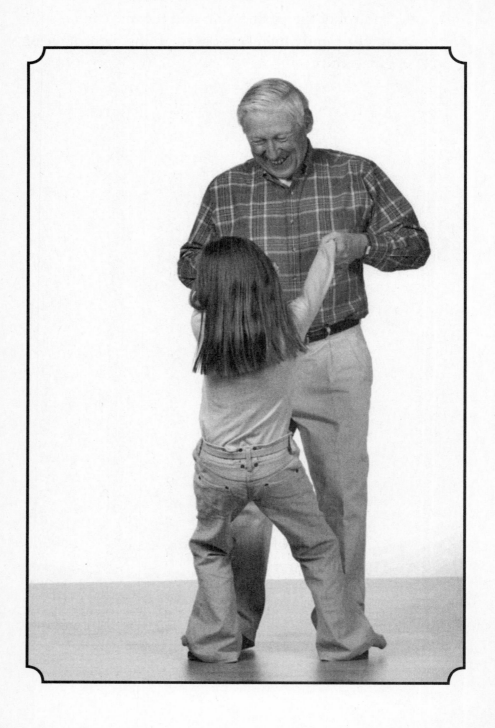

CHAPTER 9

What to Do
With Your Home

Your home is one of your biggest assets in Medicaid because it is excluded while you are living, but can become the subject of collections when the Medicaid recipient dies. There are different tactics you can use to make sure that your home is not taken by the state when someone in the family is on Medicaid or will be applying for Medicaid.

If you are permanently in a nursing home and no relative lives in your home, you must make an effort to sell your home by listing your property with a realtor or selling it privately.

Transfer your home with a special power of appointment. Here, you would transfer the ownership of your house to someone else, while reserving your right to redirect the house to a different person at a later time. You could exercise this power during your lifetime (by a deed) or at your death (by a will), subject to certain limitations. With this tool, the state would be unable to go after the house either during your lifetime or after your death. Though, you would lose the legal right to live in the house.

Keep It, Sell It or Transfer House and Property to Kids?

This is a major question older people over 65 ask when the time comes to think about a nursing home or just passing on real estate and money to family members. Determinations should be made of the home. You can have a registered real estate agent appraise the home for value. That, at least, gives you an idea of what it is worth.

Keeping the house has its benefits in that you will have a place to live and not have to deal with an unfamiliar place. Although there is some inheritance tax, it is often not much less than income tax to be paid. The drawbacks include on death of the owner, there will be an inheritance tax on the property. If the owner becomes ill, there will be no lien and the state does not require it to be sold. Yet, upon the death of the person, the state can claim the estate of the person for the amount used for Medicaid. They cannot collect if another person owns the estate.

If you sell your home, federal income tax allows $250,000 exclusion of the gain on the sale of the principal residence. It allows $500,000 for a married couple.

The proceeds from the sale of your home can be given to the intended heir without the payment of a federal gift tax. If the donor of this money applies for medical assistance, the application must report any gifts within the five years preceding the application. This can be a serious problem because the Medicaid applicant will have no money unless the transfer took place more than five years previous to the eligibility. The older person has to live somewhere and may need to use proceeds for the rental of accommodations.

When you transfer the deed to your kids, they become liable for maintenance, taxes, and insurance. There will be no inheritance tax on the property for one year.

The gift or transfer will result in a five-year period of Medicaid ineligibility. Giving the house away and reserving the right to live there will result in an inheritance tax on the full value of the house on the date of death. Another problem with transferring the deed is that if the person dies or is involved in divorce, creditors can claim the property.

Joint Ownership

Joint ownership is when two parties own property together. The term property may apply to a residence or business. If one owner dies, the property does not have to go through probate. This often applies to real estate owned like a home by a married couple. A parent can also jointly own a home with a child.

If the parent has only one child's name on the deed for joint ownership but wants to divide the property among other children, this presents a problem. When the parent dies, the child whose name is on the joint ownership does not have to carry out the parent's wishes. He or she will be the sole owner of the property.

A remarriage can result in your children being disinherited under a joint ownership. Children's creditors may try to collect on their share of the property. Your property could end up with someone else owning it other than the person you intended. A co-owner could transfer your shares to someone else without your knowledge or approval. If anyone is in a high-risk profession, the house is subject to the risk of that profession. The gift tax and estate costs could be extremely high. It is awfully hard to remove a co-owner's name from a deed without their approval.

Joint ownership allows the surviving spouse to do whatever they want with the previously jointly owned property during their life and ultimately leave it to anyone they wish at death, regardless of your desires. This can be an issue in second and third marriages.

You can transfer the house and property to your kids, but this is a disqualifying factor when you apply for Medicaid. You will have to take the cost of your home and property and divide it by the cost of a nursing home per month in your state. This will give you the amount of time you may be disqualified from Medicaid. When you deed the house to someone, you no longer own it; the control is lost over what happens. Your kids can kick you out or make you move and even sell the property if they choose.

Add Children's Names to Deed

Adding your children's names to your deed means that they own half your home upon your death. It frees property from getting tied up in probate court.

Unless you are wealthy or use it early, it will not save you much in estate taxes. Since your children own part of the home, creditors can come after it as an asset. Once their names are on the deed, you have to have the agreement of the child to get the name off the deed. Minor children on the deed needs someone appointed by the court to represent them before you can do anything with the home. Minors cannot transfer property or refinance. You will have to pay for legal fees to get someone to represent the minors. In conclusion, do not add minor children on the deed of your home.

To get adults or minor children's names off the deed, you can file a quitclaim deed in which they say they have no interest in this house. Yet, you may run into a problem if the child wants some money from the ownership of this property. What if your child runs into drug problems or tax trouble? You may have to sell your home to settle the debt for them, which is one of the drawbacks of this type of ownership.

Transfer of Home to a Sibling

The transfer of a home to a sibling of a Medicaid applicant will not incur a penalty if the brother or sister was living in the house at least one year prior to the date the applicant was admitted to a nursing home. Another factor to remember is that the sibling has an equity interest in the house. This means that some percentage of the home was gifted to them. This can be a small amount, sometimes as little as 2 percent.

If a Medicaid applicant transfers a home to a child who is under age 21, blind, or disabled, it will not cause any penalties to the applicant. If you can prove you made the transfer of a home for reasons other than qualifying for Medicaid and the transfer falls into the five-year look-back period, it may be excused. You must present to the state clear and objective evidence that the house was transferred to the applicant for reasons other than qualifying for Medicaid.

Joint Ownership with Right of Survivorship

This means both owners own 100 percent of the asset. If a husband and wife both have names on the deed, it means you both own the entire house, not half.

The 100 percent ownership by each partner makes right of survivorship work. This can refer to bank accounts, stocks, or anything else. It delays the need to go to probate court. When a joint tenant dies, they lose all ownership rights and it passes to the person who survives. He or she cannot give away ownership to anyone through a will.

To establish ownership when one person dies, the owner simply issues and records an affidavit of death. The transfer of property is simple and inexpensive.

Transfer to Children's While Keeping Life Estate

You can transfer your house to one or more children in the house but retain your life estate. When you die, the title passes automatically to the child or children to whom you deeded the interest in the house.

You have the right to live in the house during your lifetime. After death, the estate is subject to taxes and the children who own the home will receive a stepped-up tax basis. If you are on Medicaid, the state may be able to force a sale of the property to collect the value of the life estate. After you die, the property goes to your children without going to probate court.

You can give your children 1 percent interest and own the home together as joint tenants with the right to survivorship. The transfer of 1 percent would be penalized but not worth much in taxes. It may not hurt you if you apply for Medicaid because a transfer of 1 percent is not much of a gift. If you decide to use joint tenants, consult an experienced lawyer who is familiar and experienced with Medicaid law.

Life Estates

A life estate is a form of interest in a piece of property that allows the owner to retain full interest in the property until his or her death, but gives legal title to another person. You can purchase a life estate in your child's home if you move in, for instance.

If a parent sells his or her home and moves into the home of an adult child, a life estate can be another way to protect the parent's assets. The child signs a deed transferring a percent of their home equal to the amount of the parent's estate, and the parent transfers cash to the child in the amount equal to the value of that interest. They must live in the house at least one year after the deed is signed; otherwise, purchase of interest is called a gift to the child. Medicaid can count it.

Here is an example: Jane and Ted purchased a home for $700,000. Ted's mother, Mary, has declining health and needs assistance during the day. She sells her home and moves in with Jane and Ted, writing them a check in exchange for a life estate. If, after one year, she has to be moved to a nursing home, interest in her house will not be counted, since it is considered an interest in a personal residence and such an interest is almost always excluded as an asset.

Purchase a Joint Interest in a Child's Home

Sometimes, parents will purchase a joint interest in the child's house. They must reside in the home at least one year before moving into a nursing home to have this valid and not counted as a gift transaction. The longer the parent resides in the home after purchasing a joint interest, the better it looks to Medicaid when someone has to apply for benefits.

This can reduce the estate tax liability and removes valuable assets from your estate, thus lowering your estate tax liability. Parents who purchase a home jointly with a child share the home's value. An alternative is a joint purchase, but not a typical joint ownership. One party purchases the life interest and the other purchases the remainder. There is no gift tax, as long as the property is valued and each party paid his or her appropriate share.

Life interest is just that, interest for life. Interest terminates at the person's death, as there is nothing to transfer and thus nothing is subject to estate taxes. Whoever owns the remainder of the interest is now the owner of the property.

In cases of joint purchase, there is nothing transferred at death. Commonly, when family members are parents to a split-interest transaction, the remainder interest is valued at zero. The purchase is deemed a gift from the life tenant to the remainder interest holder.

Child Moves into Your Home

If it so happens that your child will move into your home to provide around-the-clock care, Medicaid will allow the applicant the right to transfer the homestead to the caregiver. The rules require that the caregiver live in the homestead at least two years immediately before the admission to a long-term care facility and provided the care that would otherwise have required long-term care as documented by a physician's statement. The two-year period must be made immediately before the nursing home entry. A stay in an assisted living center would break the continuous period.

There are caregiver agreements covered by Medicaid for the elderly who need care at home and do not want to move out. There is often a relative willing to move in to care for them. Caregiver agreements are written contracts in which a relative agrees to care for someone for an agreed-upon amount. Often, the home and person will be investigated; a criminal background check may result.

Living with a parent can cause changes in the family roles. You will find it stressful and differences in sleeping, eating, and social patterns may be hard to adjust to. You should talk about the move before you do it. Be honest and look at the pros and cons. Do you want to devote the time needed to helping your family member or would you resent it?

A program in Massachusetts allows family members to stay at home and be paid to care for fragile elderly relatives who might otherwise have to go to a nursing home. Caregivers receive up to $18,000 per year for home-based care. The savings are excellent compared to the cost of a semi-private nursing home. The caregivers are supported by a team of professionals through regular home visits and telephone contact.

With help from a lawyer, Jane recently signed a contract to help an elderly aunt. She will be responsible for taking her aunt to doctor appointments, cleaning her apartment, doing her bills and helping with laundry; she is paid for her services. This service can reduce the size of an estate and eventually help the relative qualify for Medicaid assistance. It can reward the child who spends the most time caregiving, while other siblings may not have the time or the inclination to perform these duties.

Working out the terms in a contract can make the process less painful, as no one will feel as though they are being taken advantage of. The contract spells out specifically what is being done and the caregiver is compensated financially. There is an increase in this service.

Medicaid is not likely to disqualify you for having these contracts with your family. Contracts that pass the Medicaid guidelines have to follow some rules. These rules are: You cannot pay the caregiver an inflated price just to spend down assets. You can determine the current market rate for those services by contacting agencies that provide these services and getting estimates. Services can vary from meal preparation, laundry, cleaning to providing transportation. Caregivers have to pay taxes on services and only work a few hours per week. Some states offer caregiver training and education.

Parent Moves into the Home

The financial burden of taking care of an elderly parent in your home is time consuming and stressful. The pros and cons should be weighed seriously before making a commitment to caring for anyone in their home or yours. There are many factors to consider in this decision:

- Do you and your parent have a good relationship and get along? If you never did, living with them will not work for anyone. If you truly resent having to live with your elderly parent, it is better to find another alternative.

- How does the parent get along with your children and spouse or partner? These are important questions to consider before asking them to move in.

- Can you emotionally deal with becoming your parent's parent? Do your children respect the elderly person and enjoy his or her company?

- Can you include the parent in your social activities and other routines without too much stress? Does everyone in your family want the elderly person to move in? If it is just you and everyone else is against the move, you should consider other arrangements for the person.

- Most elderly relatives need care when they move in. Can you provide them with that care or find someone else to help you?

- Does your job allow you time off to take them to doctor appointments? Do you have time to take them to visit friends or the senior center where they can socialize with other people their age?

- Living arrangements are exceedingly important. Do you have the space needed to accommodate your parent? Do you have an extra room or an addition that will provide some privacy? Is it possible that you will need some special equipment like wheelchairs, walkers, grab bars in the bathroom? Do you have the money to accomplish this?

- How will their living with you work in terms of privacy and space? If you live in a small house with three children, it will not get roomier, but more crowded and congested. A larger home works better for having your elderly parent move in with you. It is important to have the space for them so they feel welcome and have some privacy. You need to set some rules so that your parent or relative respects the other members of your household.

- How safe for the elderly is your home? Do you have any loose steps or areas that need railings or ramps?

- Do you live in a steep hilly area where getting in and out of the house is difficult? Do you have an area of the house where you can go for some privacy?

- Does the parent get some assistance so he or she can contribute financially to your household and his or her own needs? How much will you have to pay out of your own pocket to help the parent live there? Will your brothers and sisters or relatives help with the financial end? Can you discuss money with your the parent so everyone knows what is expected of them?

Here are some universal rules for living with an elderly parent that apply to all families:

- Establish house rules for everyone to follow. This will help with meals, privacy, and other important issues. Set limits on both children and the elderly person so that they can get along with each other. They need to respect each other's privacy and schedules.

- Make sure everyone has some privacy. If this means adding another bathroom or having a schedule worked out, do it. If you have to rearrange the décor or buy a divider for a few rooms, do so.

- Work out a budget that includes letting the elderly person contribute to household expenses. Never assume; discuss finances before the person moves in so hidden expenses do not surprise you.

- Let the elderly person help around the house and be as independent as possible. This is good for their self-esteem. Encourage them to have their own interests and hobbies.

- If the person has health problems, keep the doctor and emergency numbers handy so that most family members know where to find them. Discuss this with your family so that when an emergency arises they will know where to look and what to do.

- Safety is important for everyone. Make sure your parent does not leave medications around if you have younger children. Toys lying around can be hazardous for anyone with walking difficulties.

Taxes on the Home

Your home should be included in your taxable estate. For anyone applying for Medicaid, owing estate taxes is not a real problem. Your estate must be over $2 million and anyone with that much money does not need Medicaid.

There is a tax rule that says if you retain the right to live in your house for the rest of your life, it will be included in your taxable estate. This causes the house to get a new income tax value equal to the date of death value of the property. This eliminates any capital gains if the house is sold immediately upon your death. The right to live in the house does not have to be in writing; it can be a verbal agreement.

CHAPTER 10

Where to Contact Your State Agency

Alabama

Alabama Medicaid Agency

501 Dexter Avenue

Montgomery, AL 36103-5624

Phone: 334-242-5000

Eligibility contact: 800-362-1504

Web site: **www.medicaid.state.al.us**

Alaska

State of Alaska Health and Social Services

Medicaid Program

P. O. Box 110640

Juneau, AK 99811-0640

Phone: 907-465-3347

Fax: 907-465-5154

Web site: **health.hss.state.ak.us/dpa/programs/medicaid**

Arizona

Arizona Healthcare Cost Containment System

801 East Jefferson Street

Phoenix, AZ 85034

Phone: 602-417-4000

In-state outside Maricopa County: 800-654-8713

Web site: **www.azahcccs.gov/Site**

Arkansas

Arkansas Medicaid

Department of Medical Services

Department of Human Services

P. O. Box 1437, Slot S401

Little Rock, AR 72203-1437

Voice: 501-682-8292

TDD: 501-682-6789

Fax: 501-682-1197

Web site: **www.medicaid.state.ar.us**

California

California.gov Department of Health

Medi-Cal California Medicaid Program

Provider Enrollment Division

P. O. Box 997413

MS Code 4704

Sacramento, CA 95899-7413

Phone: 916-323-1945

Automated phone center: 800-786-4346

Web site: **www.medi-cal.ca.gov/sitemap.asp**

Colorado

Department of Healthcare Policy and Financing

1570 Grant Street

Denver, CO 80203

Phone: 303-866-3513

Toll-free: 800-221-3943

Web site: **www.chcpf.state.co.us/default.asp**

Connecticut

State of Connecticut

Department of Social Services

25 Sigourney Street

Hartford, CT 06106-5033

Phone: 800-842-1508

Web site: **www.ct.gov/dss/cwp/view.asp?a=2353&q=305218**

Delaware

Delaware Health and Social Services

Division of Medicaid & Medical Assistance

1901 N. Du Pont Highway, Lewis Bldg.

New Castle, DE 19720

Phone: 302-255-9500

Fax: 302-255-4454

Web site: **www.dhss.delaware.gov/dhss/dmma/index.html**

District of Columbia

Department of Health

Government of the District of Columbia

825 North Capitol Street NE

Washington, DC 20002

Phone: 202-671-5000

Fax: 202-442-4788

Web site: **doh.dc.gov/doh/site/default.asp?dohNav=|**

Florida

Florida Agency For Healthcare Administration

2727 Mahan Drive

Tallahassee, FL 32308

Phone: 888-419-3456

Web site: **www.fdhc.state.fl.us/Medicaid/index.shtml**

Georgia

Georgia Department of Community Health

2 Peachtree Street

Atlanta, GA 30303

Office of Rural Health Services

502 Seventh Street South

Cordele, GA 31015-1443

Phone: 404-298-1228

Toll-free: 800-766-4456

Web site: **dch.georgia.gov/02/dch/home/0,2467,31446711,00.html**

Hawaii

State of Hawaii

Department of Human Services

Med-Quest Division

801 Dillingham Boulevard, 3rd Floor

Honolulu, HI 96817-4582

Phone: 808-587-3521 or 808-587-3540

Fax: 808-587-3543

Web site: **www.med-quest.us**

Idaho

Idaho Department of Health and Welfare

Regional Medicaid Services (including Personal Care Svcs)

1120 Ironwood Drive, Suite 102

Coeur d'Alene, ID 83814

Phone: 208-769-1567

Fax: 208-666-6856

Web site: **www.healthandwelfare.idaho.gov/site/3629/ default.aspx**

Illinois

Illinois Department of Healthcare and Family Services

Department of Human Services

100 South Grand Avenue East

Springfield, IL 62762

Phone: 217-557-1601

Web site: **www.dhs.state.il.us/page.aspx?item=32238**

Indiana

Indiana Health Coverage Program

EDS Provider Enrollment and Waiver

P. O. Box 7263

Indianapolis, IN 46207-7263

Claims/EDS Customer Assistance: 317-655-3240 or 800-577-1278

Member Services: 877-633-7353, Option 1

PA: 800-269-5720

Web site: **www.indianamedicaid.com/ihcp/index.asp**

Iowa

Iowa Department of Human Services

409 North 4th Street

Burlington, IA 52601

Phone: 319-753-4622 or 800-423-4724

Fax: 319-754-4628

Web site: **www.dhs.state.ia.us/dhs2005/dhs_homepage/index.html**

Kansas

Kansas Health Policy Authority

Landon State Office Building, Suite 900-N

900 SW Jackson Street

Topeka, KS 66612

Phone: 785-296-3981

Web site: **www.khpa.ks.gov/MedicalAssistanceProgram/default.html**

Kentucky

Kentucky Cabinet for Health and Family Services

Office of the Secretary

275 East Main Street

Frankfort, KY 40621

Phone: 502-564-5497

Fax: 502-564-9523

Web site: **chfs.ky.gov/dms**

Louisiana

Lousiana Office of Management and Finance

Medicaid (Health Services Financing)

628 N. 4th Street

P. O. Box 91030

Baton Rouge, LA 70821-9030

Phone: 225-342-5774

Fax: 225-342-3893

Web site: **www.dhh.louisiana.gov/offices/?ID=92**

Maine

Maine Department of Health and Human Services

Office of Maine Care Services

442 Civic Center Drive

11 State House Station

Augusta, ME 04333-0011

Phone: 207-287-9202

Member Services: 800-977-6740

Web site: **www.maine.gov/dhhs/bms**

Maryland

Maryland Department of Health and Mental Hygiene

201 West Preston Street

Baltimore, MD 21202

Phone: 877-463-3464

Web site: **www.dhmh.state.md.us**

Massachusetts

Health and Human Services

Office of Medicaid

One Ashburton Place

11th Floor

Boston, MA 02108

Phone: 617-573-1770

Web site: **www.mass.gov?pageID=eohhs2homepage&L=1& L0=Home&sid=Eeohhs2**

Minnesota

Minnesota Department of Human Services

Aging and Adult Services

P. O. Box 64976

St. Paul, MN 55164-0976

Phone: 651-431-2600

Fax: 651-431-7453

Web site: **www.dhs.state.mn.us/main**

Mississippi

Division of Medicaid

Sillers Building

550 High Street, Suite 1000

Jackson, MS 39201-1399

Phone: 601-359-6050

Web site: **www.dom.state.ms.us/index.html**

Missouri

Missouri Department of Social Services

221 West High Street

P. O. Box 1527

Jefferson City, MO 65102-1527

Aging Information Referral Line: 800-235-5503

Web site: **www.dss.mo.gov/fsd/msmed.htm**

Montana

Montana Department of Health and Human Services

Provider Relations Unit

P. O. Box 4936

Helena, MT 59604

Phone: 800-624-3958

Helena: 406-442-1837

Fax: 406-442-4402

Web site: **medicaidprovider.hhs.mt.gov**

Nebraska

Nebraska Department of Health and Human Services

301 Centennial Mall South

Lincoln, NE 68509

Phone: 402-471-3121

Web site: **www.hhs.state.ne.us/med/medindex.htm**

Nevada

Nevada Department of Health and Human Services

Carson City

1100 East William Street

Suite 101

Carson City, NV 89701

Phone: 775-684-3676

New Jersey

Department of Human Services

Division of Medical Assistance & Health Services

Quakerbridge Plaza

P. O. Box 712

Trenton, NJ 08625-0712

Phone: 800-356-1561

Web site: **www.state.nj.us/humanservices/index.shtml**

New Mexico

N.M. Human Services Department

2009 S. Pacheco Pollon Plaza

Sante Fe, NM 87504

Phone: 888-997-2583

Web site: **www.hsd.state.nm.us**

New York

Department of Health

Corning Tower, Empire State Plaza

Albany, NY 12237

Phone: 718-557-1399 or 877-472-8411

Web site: **www.health.state.ny.us/health_care/medicaid**

North Carolina

North Carolina Division of Medical Assistance

Division of Medical Assistance

1985 Umstead Drive

Raleigh, NC 27626

Phone: 800-688-6696 or 919-851-8888

Web site: **www.dhhs.state.nc.us/dma/publications.htm**

North Dakota

Department of Human Services

600 East Boulevard Avenue, Dept. 325

Bismarck, ND 58505-0250

Phone: 701-328-2310

Toll-free: 800-472-2622

Fax: 701-328-2359

Web site: **www.nd.gov/dhs/about/contact.html**

Ohio

Ohio Department of Job and Family Services

30 East Broad Street, 32nd Floor

Columbus, OH 43215-3414

Phone: 877-852-0010

Web site: **www.hsd.state.nm.us**

Oklahoma

Oklahoma Healthcare Authority

4545 N. Lincoln Blvd, Suite. 124

Oklahoma City, OK 73105

Phone: 405-522-7300

Web site: **www.ohca.state.ok.us**

Oregon

Department of Human Services

Oregon Health Plan

2466 SE Ladd

Portland, OR 97214

Phone: 503-731-3111

Web site: **www.oregon.gov/DHS/spwpd/hlth_ medhealthmed.shtml#overview**

Pennsylvania

Pennsylvania Department of Public Welfare

Office of Medical Assistance Programs

P. O. Box 2675

Harrisburg, PA 17105-2675

Phone: 800-766-5387

Web site: **www.dpw.state.pa.us/About/ContactDPW**

Puerto Rico

Medicaid Office of Puerto Rico and Virgin Islands

GPO Box 70184

San Juan, PR 00936

Phone: 787-725-4300

Toll-free: 877-725-4300

Rhode Island

Rhode Island Department of Human Services

600 New London Avenue

Cranston, RI 02920

Phone: 401-784-8100

Toll-free: 800-964-6211

Web site: **www.dhs.state.ri.us**

South Carolina

South Carolina Department of Health and Human Services

P. O. Box 8206

Columbia, SC 29202-8206

Phone: 803-898-2500

Medicaid beneficiaries: 888-549-0820

Web site: **www.dhhs.state.sc.us/whatsnew.htm**

South Dakota

South Dakota Department of Social Services

700 Governors Drive

Pierre, SD 57501

Phone: 605-773-3165

Web site: **dss.sd.gov**

Tennessee

Bureau of TennCare

310 Great Circle Road

Nashville, TN 37243

Phone: 800-342-3145

Web site: **www.state.tn.us/tenncare**

Texas

Texas Health and Human Resource Commission

Brown-Heatly Building

4900 N. Lamar Blvd.

Austin, TX 78751-2316

Phone: 512-424-6500

Medicaid Client Hotline: 800-252-8263

Web site: **www.hhsc.state.tx.us/Medicaid/med_info.html**

Utah

Utah Department of Health

Utah Medicaid Program

Cannon Health Building

(Main Utah Department of Health office building)

288 North 1460 West

Salt Lake City, UT

Phone: 800-662-9651

Web site: **health.utah.gov**

Vermont

Vermont Department of Children and Families

Economic Services Division

103 South Main Street

Waterbury, VT 05676-1201

Phone: 800-250-8427

Web site: **www.dsw.state.vt.us/Programs_Pages/Healthcare/
medicaid.htm**

Virginia

Virginia Department of Medical Assistance

600 East Broad Street

Richmond, VA 23219

Phone: 804-726-7000 (Richmond)

Toll-free: 800-552-3431

Web site: **www.dmas.virginia.gov**

Washington

Washington State Department of Social and Health Services

DSHS Constituent Services

P. O. Box 45130

Olympia, WA 98504-5130

Phone: 800-737-0617 (Washington State information only)

Web site: **fortress.wa.gov/dshs/maa**

West Virginia

West Virginia Health and Human Resources

Bureau for Medical Services

Office of Medicaid Managed Care, Room 251

350 Capitol Street

Charleston, WV 25301-3708

Phone: 304-558-6006

Web site: **www.wvdhhr.org/bms**

Wisconsin

Wisconsin Department of Health and Family Services

1 W. Wilson Street

Madison, WI 53703

Phone: 608-266-1865

Web site: **dhfs.wisconsin.gov/contact.htm**

Wyoming

ACS Wyoming Medicaid

Qwest Building

6101 Yellowstone Road, Suite 210

Cheyenne, WY 82002

Phone: 307-772-8401

Toll-free: 800-251-1268

Medicaid News from State to State

An Overview of Medicaid Laws and Programs and Some Alternative Options in Different States

Alabama

In 2007, Alabama instituted the Medicaid Personal Choices Program, an option for individuals who are part of the Elderly and Disabled waiver program. This program promotes independent living for the elderly and disabled individuals. Under this program, the person is provided a monthly allowance to hire someone to help with his or her care. They are given the power to choose their own healthcare providers and services. Participants can use the money to buy supplies, equipment, household services, and make repairs to their homes.

A new law was signed that requires all Medicaid prescription drugs to be written on tamper-resistant paper. This was because some health providers abused the system. A leading company, Medi-Scripts, provides this type of product to providers in Alabama and other states. The problem with this new law is that many physicians do not use tamper-resistant paper and never have. This law has been delayed in many states due to this fact.

The state received a $7.6 million dollar grant to transform the Medicaid paper process into an efficient, coordinated, and cost effective one. The project, called Together for Quality, was selected from 130 proposals submitted by 40 states. It seeks to create a statewide electronic health information system. The system will link Medicaid with state health agencies, providers, and private-pay clients. It will establish an effective, linked health information network.

The state expects the new computer network system to provide physicians, pharmacists, and healthcare providers information they need to improve the coordination of patient care and prevent complications. The system will help to reduce patient errors through electronic health records and increase the use of generic prescription drugs.

In Alabama during 2008, to qualify for Medicaid through SSI, the aged, blind, or disabled individual income limit cannot exceed $657 per month and $976 for a couple. For an individual, the resources limit cannot exceed $2,000 per month or $3,000 per couple. For nursing home institutionalized Medicaid, the income limit for an individual is $1,911 per month. For the Home and Community-based Waiver Program in Alabama, the income limit for the elderly and disabled is $1,911 per month, with the income resource limit being $2,000.

Alaska

Alaska reported that nationwide audits of Medicaid would begin in winter 2008. The Payment Error Rate Measurement will review how accurately all 50 states are billing Medicaid. It is a big audit for Alaska, as it will look at all Medicaid healthcare providers. States audited that have errors could face stiff penalties. Potential penalties could mean less money for Alaska Medicaid programs and other states. Each year, Alaska pays more than $1 million in medical costs. State and federal lawmakers having to make budget cuts have asked for these audits to help determine if Medicaid runs efficiently. The Center for Medicare and Medicaid will randomly examine claims that Alaska has submitted. The audit begins January 2008, looking at bills submitted since October 2007. The results are expected at the end of 2009.

Affiliated Computer Services will be involved in building the management information system for Alaska Medicaid. The contract is for ten years and may be worth about $130 million. The Dallas-based business will develop claims processing, a call center for client support, a pharmacy support network, and operational support for the Medicaid system. They want to replace the old computer system, which cannot keep up with the claims filed. It will simplify electronic billing and payment for doctors.

Arizona

The role of Tribal Relations in Arizona is to be an advocate and liaison for healthcare for the American Indian; other states have similar programs to this. The person who is the liaison works with 22 Arizona Indian tribes and three health services. They also work with urban Indian health programs and stakeholder organizations. The state has a separate list of medical providers that treat this special population. They are trained to be sensitive to their special needs. Older American Indians can get healthcare through Medicaid and other government programs in this state.

One of the programs for seniors in this state is Medicare Cost Sharing, which is for people 65 years or older and the blind or disabled. There is no limit on resources, but applicants must be eligible for Medicare Part A, which is the hospital program. There are special income limits on this program. For qualified Medicare Beneficiaries, the monthly income limit for individuals is $851 and $1,144 for couples. Benefits are payments of Part A and B premiums, deductibles, and co-insurance. A Specified Low Income Medicare Beneficiary must be receiving Medicare Part B and the monthly income must fall between $851 and $1,021 for individuals and $1,369 to $1,444.01 for couples. The benefit is payment of the Medicare Part B premium. A Qualified Individual monthly income must be $1,012 through $1,149 for individuals and $1,369 to $1,541 for couples. The benefit is also payment of Medicare Part B Premium.

Another program is SSI, or Medical Assistance Only, which is for individuals 65 or older, and the blind or disabled. Qualified participants should not receive any money from Supplemental Security Income Program. The monthly income limit is $851 for an individual and $1,414 for a couple. The good news is that there is no limit for resources or property.

The Arizona Long-term Care System is another program for the elderly over 65 years old, and blind or disabled individuals. Program participants do not have to be in a nursing home, as many live in their own homes. They should need care at a nursing facility level. Some participants live in assisted living centers. The program covers medical care, doctor's office visits, hospitalization, prescriptions, lab work, and behavioral health services. The monthly income limit for this program is $1,119 a month and the resource limit is $2,000 for single individuals. If the person has a spouse who resides in the community, that person can keep half of the couple's resources, or up to $104,000.

Arkansas

Due to a change in the law on January 1, 2006, the state of Arkansas can no longer cover prescription drugs under Medicaid if the patient is eligible for both. It will only pay for prescriptions under Medicare Part D. These patients are called dual eligibles.

To get full Medicaid benefits in Arkansas, you should be 65 years or older. You can also be under the age of 19, blind, disabled, living in a nursing home, or have a medical need of home and community-based services. A program called Medicaid Spend-Down is for clients who have too much money, but are spending most of it on healthcare. This program allows you to qualify for Medicaid anyway. You must apply to the program every three months to be evaluated for eligibility.

The Elder Choices Program provides in-home services to those 65 and over who meet the medical and financial criteria. The program prevents the elderly person from going into a nursing home by providing services for them in the community.

Adult Companion is a new service that allows the elderly person to have a person help with meals, laundry, cleaning, bathing, eating, dressing and personal hygiene. The program is for therapeutic medical purposes. Adult daycare provides care for functionally impaired adults. Services include meals, transportation, and recreational activities. Adult Day Healthcare is a program of continuous care available to some elderly patients in Arkansas. It includes chores and other services including home-delivered meals, homemaker services, chores, and respite care.

California

Financial problems stemming from Med-Cal payment errors and the recent Medicare audit caused the Kingsburg District Hospital to close their emergency room service doors. They do not plan to reopen the emergency room even if the payment errors are resolved. Officials report that Med-Cal owes the hospital $275,000 due to an error; they hope to receive the reimbursement soon. Medicare is withholding payments due to a problem in an audit performed. Local nursing homes have joined the hospital in criticizing the Medicare audits. Medicare has denied money for claims for rehabilitation hospitals.

One program for Med-Cal of California is the Assisted Living Waiver pilot program. It provides those qualified with an alternative to living in nursing homes. There are two types of assisted living center residences available: one is a residential care facility for the elderly; the other is publicly subsidized housing. This program allows the elderly person to live in a community setting rather than a long-term nursing home. It is offered in three counties: Sacramento, San Joaquin, and Los Angeles. Some of the benefits of the program include skilled nursing transition assistance, community transition assistance, and consumer education.

The In Home Supportive Service Plus program in California provides the aged, blind, and disabled with a wide variety of services for personal care. Applicants must meet medical and financial requirements, and need help to remain in their home independently. The program provides domestic services, meal preparation, routine laundry assistance, personal care services, food shopping, transportation to medical appointments, and heavy cleaning.

The Multi Purpose Senior Services program provides home and community-based services to those over 65 and disabled as an alternative to nursing homes. It is for Med-Cal participants who need nursing level care, but who want to remain at home. Services provided include case management, personal care, respite care, transportation, housing assistance, adult daycare, and meal services.

The Nursing Facility Acute Hospital Waiver was renamed on January 1, 2007. This program combines three other community-based waiver programs. It is supposed to provide Med-Cal beneficiaries with acute medical conditions the option of returning to their home or community to live after hospitalization. The program provides a safe transition from the medical facility to the community or home for patients. They must also provide home services to those in danger of needing long-term nursing care.

The Program of All Inclusive Care for the Elderly (PACE) offers medical, social, and long-term care services. They use adult daycare health services as one of the primary ways of delivering services to clients. Individuals must be 55 years or older and live in the program area. Participants receive payments from Medicare and Medicaid, and the program also takes private-pay clients.

The governor of California proposed a $1.1 million dollar cut in Med-Cal for 2008. Since the program receives federal matching dollars, the loss of funds could total about $2 billion dollars. He proposed that families must prove eligibility for programs four times during the year. Currently, they only have to provide proof of yearly income once a year. The new rule is expected to save the state $92 million dollars.

The University of California at Merced was looking for a site for a telemedicine center for poor and disadvantaged patients who did not have access to medical specialists. Videoconferencing equipment in this new center will allow someone sitting in the center to be diagnosed by someone 80 to 90 miles away. It would be located in either San Francisco or Davis. This is part of a project to design four health centers that will serve the state's uninsured population. The intent is to work with clinics committed to telemedicine. The project has more than $1 million in funding.

Colorado

Medicaid is available to low-income individuals 65 years old and over who need healthcare and long-term care. The income limit is $637 for individuals and $937 for couples for 2008. Resource limits are less than $2,000 for individuals and $3,000 for couples in this state.

Limits for Medicaid are as follows: individuals who are over the age of 60 with an income less than $662 per month and $1,325 for couples; the resources limit must be less than $2,000 per individual and $3,000 for couples. Some applicants are eligible for the Old Age Pension (OAP), a program funded by the state of Colorado. OAP recipients receive some health benefits similar to Medicaid for physician visits, hospital care, and prescription drugs.

Often, the elderly need home care or services, but do not have the money to pay for it. In 2008, individuals with income less than $1,911 and resources less than $2,000 could qualify for HCBS. They must meet the financial guidelines and need assistance with bathing, eating, or dressing. Those who are a danger to others and need supervision or are incontinent may be eligible for Medicaid in assisted living or nursing homes.

There is proposed legislation for 2008 to address the issue of elderly individuals who have enough income to pay for long-term care before they become eligible for Medicaid. The legislation wants to limit the amount that someone can put in a pooled trust. The source of funding for this type of trust may be limited to personal injury settlements and retroactive Social Security payments.

A new telehealth center opened in Craig for veterans offering on-site nursing care and videoconferencing with doctors. The Craig Community VA Telehealth Clinic will service more than 600 veterans in Colorado and Wyoming. It will be a prototype for other clinics to be designed.

Connecticut

Connecticut is receiving a $24.2 million grant called Money Follows the Person. The purpose is to use the money to give the elderly person more flexibility in their living arrangements. The grant will help fund 24-hour care so applicants can live at home instead of going into a nursing home. The program plans to move some elderly patients from the nursing home back into the community. The grant covers 24-hour care such as live-in assistance, personal management, and making changes to the home to make it accessible for fragile elderly clients. Joe Santiago initiated the program in the state because he wanted to bring his elderly mother home to live with him.

Medicaid funding will be increased from 50 to 75 percent with the success of the state's program. The Connecticut Home Care Program for Elders will include personal care assistance and assisted living plans for 2008. The Connecticut Home Care Program for Elders is available to anyone 65 years or older at risk of having to go to a nursing home. They must meet the strict financial and medical eligibility requirements. This program may help the elderly continue to live at home. Benefits include care management services, adult health daycare, chore services, companion services, home-delivered meals, homemaker services, and personal care attendants.

Delaware

The state Division of Medicaid and Medical Assistance in Delaware provides several long-term care programs for the elderly. Medicaid Nursing Facility Care is a program geared to the elderly who need long-term nursing home care. They must meet eligibility requirements and need long-term medical care. They must be Medicaid eligible and willing to live in a nursing home.

The Elderly Home and Community Based Waiver services provide case management for those determined to live at home. The services must be monitored for quality and use contracted healthcare providers. The Personal Care program is for persons 18 to 59 years old who meet the medical criteria. Funding comes from Medicaid, state funds, the Older American Act, and the Social Services Block Grant. Services such as bathing, meal preparation, and housekeeping help a person to remain living independently. Adult Day Services is a program for individuals 60 years and older. There are approximately six to seven individual daycare centers that have this program. These centers provide care for the elderly while family members are at work.

The Personal Emergency Response System program is for those who live alone or elderly adults with disabilities. It is a device that helps a person get medical help immediately by pushing a button connected to their phone that dials the hospital or center. Trained personnel at the center assist the elderly person with emergency medical help. Institutional or Respite Care is for those 60 years or older with physical disabilities. Respite care can be arranged for the caregiver on a weekly or other basis depending on the circumstances. There are different types of respite care available for these services.

The Nursing Home Transition program is a state-funded program that plans to identify, inform, and assist nursing home residents who are Medicaid eligible with the option to move into a community setting. Programs offer case management to accomplish this goal. Any resident of a nursing home is eligible if found medically able to participate.

Florida

Florida is trying to make some major changes with Medicaid. The governor has proposed that Medicaid recipients be able to buy their own healthcare coverage from managed care organizations and other private medical networks. This would be the first state to allow private companies to determine the scope of Medicaid programs for the elderly, disabled, and children. This is one of the state's first efforts in 2008 to cut Medicaid's soaring costs. Florida plans on introducing managed care without any restrictions, allowing private companies to decide who will be covered and for what services. This gives private companies the power to determine treatment of low-income patients.

Under this plan, those eligible would qualify for a set amount of money each month. It would rise and fall depending on their medical needs. The money would be used to pay premiums for managed care, insurance programs, or providers. The private companies used would be able to set up competitive pricing. The competition between the companies would hold down medical costs. The state would offer more money for services to those who live healthier lives, like flexible spending accounts. Florida would monitor companies to make sure they could deliver medical services needed, counsel Medicaid applicants as to which service was best for each person, and set spending levels for the program. The plan involves many elderly and poor clients in the program.

The Assisted Living for the Elderly waiver program is a home- and community-based effort in Florida. It covers case management, assisted living, and incontinence supplies. The assisted living option includes attendant care, chores, behavior management, companion services, intermittent nursing, medication administration, personal care, physical therapy, and speech therapy. It is available for individuals ages 60 to 65 years old and determines who is disabled according to Social Security standards. The person must require assistance with four or more activities of daily living. They must have a diagnosis from a physician of dementia or Alzheimer's disease, or another degenerative or chronic disease.

Georgia

The state of Georgia has a coalition of professional groups that have joined together to address Medicaid underpayment to physicians. These organizations are chambers of commerce, businesses, healthcare providers, and county governments. Healthcare providers complain that every year they are asked to cover more medical treatments for less and less money; some hospitals blame the Medicaid system for the budget shortage. State money exceeds the federal funding by a 2 to 1 ratio. Providers say that by failing to reimburse the low-income families, the state is wasting the Medicaid dollar. They want to increase payment to Medicaid providers by more than $40 million. Another goal is to maximize the federal matching dollars for Medicaid, leaving no money on the table. The final goal is to pay all Georgia Medicaid healthcare providers reasonable costs by 2011. This group is called ACCESS (Community Coalition for Effective Sustainable Success). They threaten that many physicians will have to stop treating Medicaid patients due to the low reimbursement rates. It is not a decision that most physicians want to make, but sometimes it is a necessity to survive financially.

The Georgia Medicaid Management Program is for the aged, blind, and disabled. The program provides patients with a 24-hour registered nurse hotline. The nurse will talk with clients and work with them to help educate them about their illness and treatment. The hotline nurse will talk with the client's doctor to see how she can assist each client with the doctor's specific treatment plan. The nurse will discuss medications and how to take them properly to reduce side effects, and also diet and exercise. This service also provides free education about health issues and a newsletter.

The Georgia Better Healthcare program matches the Medicaid members to a primary care physician or provider. The key point of the program is to improve access to medical care, especially for primary care providers. They hope to reduce the unnecessary use of medical services. Managed care, instead of a fee for service benefits, is directed toward a specific network of hospitals and doctors.

The average cost of a nursing home in Georgia is $4,257.60; this is an income cap state. The state has expanded its definition of estate recovery, so more assets may be countable. The home equity limit is $500,000, and Medicaid will not cover long-term care for individuals with equity above this limit.

The Medicaid Estate Recovery Program can put a lien on the Medicaid recipients' homes after paying benefits to them for six months. After the recipient's death, the state will try to collect on the lien so it can be reimbursed for the health coverage. This can mean forcing the sale of the home to collect what is owed, or this can be waived if a spouse or dependent child is living in the home. In addition, an estate valued at $25,000 or less will not be subject to estate recovery.

Hawaii

Hawaii has home and community-based waiver programs. One program is called Nursing Homes Without Walls, which provides services for elderly individuals at home. PACE is a managed care program for the elderly, age 55 or over, who live in urban Honolulu. Normally, the elderly person must be 65 or older and in need of long-term care to qualify for this program.

The Medicaid Fee For Service program is the traditional Medicaid program for low-income Hawaiian residents 65 years or older. It covers long-term care in nursing homes and some home and community services to those that meet the financial and legal requirements. Some Medicaid long-term care patients may have a lien put on their homes for their payments back to the state.

Quest Adult Coverage Expansion Program gives those not covered by Medicaid and the uninsured coverage for many medical services needed like doctor visits, prescription drugs, and hospital stays.

The Residential Alternative Community Care Program provides long-term care services to adults in assisted living centers and similar facilities.

Idaho

Personal Care is a program for the aged with a disability or the elderly with traumatic brain injuries who need assistance to remain at home. The program provides services such as housekeeping, transportation, personal grooming, transportation, and more.

Unisys Corporation signed a seven-year contract with the Idaho Department of Health and Welfare to deliver financial and operational support for the state's Medicaid program. They upgraded and designed a Medicaid management information system for the state. The Health PAS system is a commercial software program that processes unlimited payments and claims, and provides medical service authorization, call center support, and management.

Recently, the state awarded Thomas Healthcare a multiyear contract to provide healthcare decision support and data warehousing. They plan to use their DSS/DW system to manage the $9 million healthcare claims submitted to their Medicaid program. The company hopes to help the state fight fraud and manage costs.

Illinois

Illinois Cares Rx Plus provides prescription assistance to seniors 65 or older who have an annual income of $23,225 for individuals and $31,264 for couples. It helps those with or without Medicare who need medicine. It covers almost all prescription drugs. Illinois Care Rx Basic covers anyone 65 year or older with disabilities. The income level for individual is $24,808, $32,916 for couples, and $41,023 for families. It covers prescription drugs that treat ten common diseases, including Alzheimer's, arthritis, cancer, diabetes, and glaucoma.

Illinois developed the Supportive Living Program as an alternative to nursing homes. It is for low-income elderly people and those with disabilities under Medicaid. It combines apartment-style housing with personal care services so residents can live as independently as possible. The program pays for home care services, but the person must pay rent. The state also has the PACE program for the elderly 55 and older.

Indiana

In 2007, the state Family and Social Services Administration negotiated two managed care contracts for state Medicaid beneficiaries who are blind, elderly, or disabled. They account for about two-thirds of Medicaid applicants. They cost the state about $3 billion annually.

The state has a Medicaid Waiver program that allows it to enroll low-income residents in a subsidized high-deductible care program similar to a health savings account. To qualify, applicants must be less than 200 percent of the federal poverty level. Beneficiaries make payments similar to a personal and wellness responsibility account, not exceeding 5 percent of the family income. The account deductible is $1,100. Once the applicant reaches the deductible, the private insurance purchased takes effect. Health benefits include physician consultation, prescription drugs, home health services, and inpatient and outpatient care, mental health, and substance abuse treatment.

The state is trying to make primary care the focus of the Medicaid program. The Indiana Check Up Plan provides increased payments and bonuses to primary care providers who participate in the Medicaid program. They have approved a rate increase of 25 percent or $32 million annually for primary care doctors. This includes preventive care, evaluation and management, and early periodic screening. The state is trying to get to a value-driven healthcare system. The system has not seen a raise in 14 years.

Iowa

The home and community-based waiver programs are for older citizens who may need help so that they can stay at home and live independently. Participants must be eligible for Medicaid and meet certain requirements.

There are seven different programs; not all apply to the elderly. The HCBS Elderly Waiver program is for seniors 65 years or older who need assistance. It covers adult daycare, case management, help with chores, home-delivered meals, homemaker services, nursing care, nutritional counseling, respite, senior companions, and transportation.

The HCBS II and Handicapped IH Waiver are for seniors 65 years and older who are blind or disabled. This program provides adult daycare, attendant care, homemaker services, nursing services, home health aides, respite care, nutritional counseling, personal emergency response, and other services.

In 2007, Iowa sued about 78 drug companies on the grounds of inflating costs of drugs to Medicaid customers. The state lost billions of dollars due to manufacturers inflating prices to get a larger share of the market. The lawsuit covers a 13-year period. The state hopes to recover the money lost.

Wal-Mart in the state of Iowa was the largest employer of workers who received Medicaid benefits. They had 845 workers who were getting Medicaid benefits while employed for the store. Other companies who had employees receiving Medicaid benefits were Tyson Fresh Meats, Casey's General Stores, and Hy-Vee Inc. Critics say that the state is allowing companies to pay low wages and not offer adequate health insurance. Medicaid is designed for those in poverty and not working.

Kansas

Kansas will upgrade its Medicaid Management Information System under a six-year contract with EDS (Electronic Data Systems) for $160 million. The project is outsourced, meaning another company handles the work for the state, and the company will take over the enrollment for Medicaid and the children's program in the state.

The Statewide Independence Council of Kansas supports a nursing home bed tax as a way to raise money for the HCBS waiver program for the elderly. Every bed in a nursing home would be taxed the rate now is $2 per day. The money raised would be used to pay for home based community services for the elderly that stay at home and other 50 percent would cover the cost of increased nursing home care. This is The Statewide Independent Living Council of Kansas.

Kentucky

KyHealth Choices is a new name for the state's Medicaid program. It is designed to stretch the program to meet the needs of the population it serves. It encourages the clients to be responsible for their own healthcare. It serves the elderly and disabled, who often fall into the same category. Some of the programs covered since 2007 are listed below.

The Self Directed Program under the HCBS program hopes to provide community services to individuals at home. Participants are able to control the services by choosing the services they need to live at home. It will serve more than 200 individuals in different parts of the state who need help, including the elderly. Goods and Services is another component that helps individuals reduce the need for services by purchasing goods and services that promote the independence of the applicants at home.

In May 2007, the state was awarded a Money Follows the Person

Rebalancing Demonstration Grant. The amount of the grant was for $49,831,530 to provide money to help seniors move from nursing homes back into the community with family or foster care. Any Medicaid applicant who is in a nursing home for more than six months is eligible for the program. Elderly clients are included in the target populations served by the grant.

The state has an Adult Daycare and Alzheimer's Respite Program. It provides social and related services for the elderly with the disease. Participants must be 60 years old, fragile, and in need of care during the day. They must be experiencing mental confusion and need care for nutrition and preventive services that assist them from injuring themselves. The program monitors taking medication properly and some other medical services. Applicants must be diagnosed by a physician to have dementia or Alzheimer's disease. This qualifies them for the adult daycare services, adult healthcare services, or respite care for caregivers.

Kentucky made efforts to cut Medicaid spending by offering more benefits to patients that follow disease management programs. Someone who keeps up with treatments for diabetes could earn credits for dental or vision care. The program was split into four separate programs that covers different groups of people. It offers a program for elderly clients covered by Medicare as part of the Medicaid program.

More than 1,000 disabled Medicaid users gathered to ask the state not to cut Medicaid benefits. They claimed that cutting benefits to physically and mentally disabled members would not necessarily save the state money. Cutting the Medicaid budget might mean federal matching grants would be cut.

For every 30 cents the state pays on Medicaid, the federal government spends 70 cents.

The EDS Corporation won a $170 million contract to design a management information system for Kentucky in 2007. The system will have financial services, claim processing, a call center, data storing, mail room, and provider training. The new system will allow Medicaid recipients to submit claims in a variety of different electronic formats. The new system is expected to serve 691,000 Medicaid users and over 35,000 healthcare providers.

Despite budget cuts, the state of Kentucky has no plans to cut Medicaid spending. Only modest increases were proposed in the current program. More than 722,000 residents will continue to receive coverage under the program. To avoid cuts in the face of escalating healthcare costs, the governor proposed to increase spending by 3 percent in 2008 and 7 percent in 2009. That money will increase the budget for Medicaid.

Fraud in Medicaid is a problem in all states. The state of Kentucky encourages anyone who knows of anyone ripping off the system to report it. Health fraud is anyone misrepresenting information intentionally to qualify for Medicaid benefits or Medicare. Fraud is also a doctor or provider billing for services never performed. Potential violators are many physicians, healthcare providers, and hospitals, laboratories that process tests for doctors, billing services, or even Medicaid recipients themselves. Anyone can report fraud by calling the Kentucky Office of Inspector General at (1-800-372-2970.) The mailing address is:

Cabinet For Healthcare and Family Services

Office of the Inspector General Division
of Special Investigations

275 East Main Street, 5 E-D

Frankfort, KY 40621

Kentucky Medicaid will reimburse for the purchase of durable medical equipment under the Durable Medical Equipment Program. This is defined as any equipment used to serve a medical purpose. Some of the items covered are wheelchairs, hospital beds, orthodontic appliances, prosthetic devices, and disposable medical equipment ordered by the provider that deems it usable in the home.

Louisiana

The number of uninsured adults and children since 2005 have been steadily declining in the state of Louisiana due to the aftermath of Hurricane Katrina. The adult rate dropped from 24 percent in 2005 to 21.2 percent in 2007. The changes are due to losses and changes in the population due to Hurricanes Katrina and Rita.

During 2007, the Elderly and Disabled Adult waiver program added about 1,500 new people to the program. The program now has 4,403 persons who receive assistance at home. This helps the elderly persons who would otherwise be in a nursing home to receive care at home. They must meet the medical and income guidelines.

The state received a $15.9 million grant from the Federal Communications Commission and Health and Hospital Department for 109 hospitals to get a new medical management information system. The grant provides the hospitals with money to upgrade Internet connections to increase speed and efficiency of processing information. The money will buy the hardware and software needed to upgrade the systems and connections. This will be an asset in the event of another disaster like Hurricane Katrina. Doctors in one part of the state could transmit patient information much more quickly. If many patients left their homes without paperwork, as they did when Hurricane Katrina struck, the computer system will have the information available, allowing them to continue medical treatment without interruption.

The state received a $30.9 million grant for home- and community-based services for people with disabilities and the elderly who need long-term care. These services will help reduce the state's need for institutional care, and gives residents a choice of home- and community-based services, instead of just entering a nursing home. The state received $524,000 the first year for administrative and startup costs. The rest of the money will be distributed to the state over a five-year period. The grant is under the Money Follows the Person rebalancing program, which seeks to shift nursing home residents back into the community.

The key components of the grant include that it provides those applicants for Medicaid money for services in a setting of their choice. It ensures that those who move into the community will receive home- and community-based services. The federal government will pay 75 to 90 percent of the cost of moving a nursing home resident out of the facility and back into the community. This will be done through a 50 percent higher than usual Medicaid match rate for qualified applicants' expenditures.

The Department of Health and Hospital received two grants

totaling $56 million to restore access to healthcare in the hard-hit Hurricane Katrina regions of Greater New Orleans. The Professional Workforce Supply Grant of $35 million will go towards licensing and retaining healthcare professionals in that area. They hope to employ 600 and more from this grant in the areas of Orleans, Jefferson, St. Bernard, and Plaquemine. It will be used to attract physicians, internists, dentists, registered nurses, pediatricians, and psychiatrists.

The Providers Stabilization Grant, worth $26.2 million, will be used to make payments to healthcare facilities that have financial burdens after the disaster. The grant will benefit hospitals, skilled nursing homes, psychiatric and community mental health centers.

Maine

The Maine governor said that Medicaid cuts would have a disastrous impact on children and venerable populations like the elderly. These changes are short-sighted and will increase costs in the long run. If these new rules are imposed, they will damage not only the citizens but also the healthcare sector of the economy. It would be difficult for Maine to replace the federal funding they received for the many Medicaid programs.

Maine would have to cut $70 million in health and human services to balance the budget. This would include reductions in homemaking services for the elderly that could put some in nursing homes. The governor said vulnerable people would be hurt and there is no way to get around this. Medicaid serves the state's poorest elderly. It is mostly state-funded with no matching federal grants. The cuts include a $700,000 reduction in Medicaid homemaker services to help the elderly with grocery shopping, cooking, laundry, and housekeeping. There are 376 people on the waiting list seeking these services.

Eliminations of $700,000 for independent living projects for low-income fragile elderly in government subsidized rents is another problem. One village impacted would be Larrabee Village in Westbrook, Maine, with more than 150 tenants. Approximately $400,000 will be cut from adult daycare that provides meal, social activities, and transportation for those living at home. Elimination of funding for training, respite, and support for caregivers of families dealing with Alzheimer's disease is included. There is a $3.3 million reduction in payments to boarding homes for seniors by eliminating bed hold days when a resident is not at home. The cut of home-based services will force many elderly people into nursing homes or more expensive treatment programs.

The number of low-income residents is higher in Maine than in many other states. Approximately 21 percent of the elderly are over 65 years old and on Medicaid, compared to 14 percent in other states nationally. Additionally, Maine has the second-highest cost per Medicaid recipient in the country. The state could save $1 million if it had average spending for everyone on the program. Maine enrolls more people in Medicaid than is funded by federal money. It offers a more generous benefit package than most states.

An audit by the U. S. Department of Health and Human Services revealed that Maine over-billed the Medicaid program by more than $44 billion in 2002 and 2003. Maine says the audit applied new billing rules not in effect at the time the billing was done. They said they will appeal the audit and do not owe the federal government money. The audit did not charge the state with fraud, but with sloppy bookkeeping and tracking claim methods. The audit said the state billed for direct services and administrative costs that were not eligible for reimbursement by Medicaid.

One major change for the Maine Medicaid system is case management, which determines how an individual's medical, social, and educational needs will be met. By limiting what can be included in case management, the program leaves the state in the position of having to cut programs that elderly people depend on.

Dan lives in Larabee Village in Maine. He is 88 years old and has almost died twice. An on-call resident assistant saved his life when he knocked the phone off the hook with his fist one time when he was suffering from a mini-stroke; Medicaid pays for these services. Many elderly residents who live in every state depend on the services funded by Medicaid. The cuts will hurt them all.

Maryland

Maryland could lose up to $75 million in federal money for case management, which is designed to provide preventive healthcare. This could affect over 200,000 state residents. The Governor says every case management program in the state will be affected by the cuts. Maryland spends a total of $150 million on case management services, with about half of this money coming from federal funding. The new rules will shift the program onto the states to keep the program intact.

The Maryland Medicaid waiver program serves the elderly, and mentally and physically ill persons. It covers a broad range of community-based services as an alternative to institutionalization. Nursing facility care may be available for those who are elderly, physically disabled, or cognitively impaired.

The Money Follows the Person Demonstration program is set for 2007 in Maryland, and runs until 2011. It is for elderly and other disabled individuals in nursing homes, intermediate care facilities, chronic care hospitals, and public institutions for mental disease who want to leave the setting and live in the community. The state plans on running an aggressive program of identifying and assisting applicants with the transition. The state hopes to have at least 2,916 individuals in the program. Transition services will include help in finding affordable housing and community-based services to help the person live independently.

HealthChoice is the name of Maryland's statewide managed care program that began in 1997. It provides healthcare to most Medicaid recipients. Eligible Medicaid recipients enroll in a managed care organization of their choice and select a primary care provider to oversee their medical program.

An MCO (Managed Care Organization) is a healthcare entity that provides services to Medicaid recipients in Maryland. There are currently seven MCOs in Maryland. The Medicaid program makes payments to the MCOs at fixed capitalization rates. Payment are often based on an applicant's past Medicaid medical records, charging higher rates for the most chronically ill and less for healthy applicants. Check with your state agency for more information about eligibility.

The Program for All Inclusive Care For the Elderly (PACE) is a comprehensive medical and social service program for fragile elderly. It is administered by the Center for Medicaid and Medicare. It assists the elderly, 55 years and older, who want to live in the community. Participants must be able to live safely in the community with home-based assistance.

The Medicaid Nursing Home Program in Maryland has 240 nursing homes enrolled in the program. Applicants must meet Medicaid financial and medical qualifications. Frequently, someone must need 24-hour supervision to qualify. Maryland pays different nursing home rates to different facilities, based on the operating cost and type of care needed.

Massachusetts

Massachusetts was awarded $2.4 million dollars in a FYO grant to community-based organizations to help identify people eligible to be enrolled in the Medicaid program. The nonprofit and healthcare organizations know the needs of their clients. They know the criteria and enrollment procedures for MassHealth. They will be a welcome asset in identifying those who need medical assistance.

Clients in MassHealth Programs who are experiencing financial hardship can apply for a hardship waiver or reduction on their premium. MassHealth will then send the applicant a waiver request form that must be returned in two weeks. Conditions that meet the hardship waiver are homelessness, 30 days late in rent or mortgage payments, facing eviction or foreclosure, medical or dental expenses,

The attorney general recovered $26.7 million in Medicaid

fraud for Massachusetts in 2007, the largest amount ever recovered. One suit was against a medical laboratory in Lynn that paid over $8.5 million to settle allegations of overpayment and inappropriate referrals. Another recovery was from a national drug company who manufactures a painkiller called OxyContin. It was ruled that the company engaged in improper marketing of the drugs to patients.

Another thirteen drug companies were found guilty of false price reporting or inflating the cost to be reimbursed more than was allowed by Medicaid.

More than 250 Massachusetts doctors have signed an open letter to the United States, warning that the health reform model in Massachusetts is failing. They believe a single-payer program is the solution to this problem. In 2006, the state designed a law that required all residents to have health insurance. An agency was created to make sure all uninsured individuals had access to health insurance. If those that did not have insurance did not purchase it, they could face a fine. Low-income residents were offered subsidies to help them buy insurance and expanded Medicaid insurance products. Money that paid for free healthcare for the poor was shifted into insurance plans. Only 37 percent of the 657,000 uninsured have gained coverage through the new system. Money that went directly to hospitals and healthcare clinics for the poor now goes through insurance companies. That is an example of a misuse of Medicaid dollars.

The Massachusetts health insurance model program has some of the following criteria: requirement for all residents to obtain health insurance as long as it is affordable; expanded insurance subsidies for residents making less than three times the federal poverty level; new penalties to punish employers who do not offer insurance to employees.

Michigan

In 2007, the Michigan state senate approved a Medicaid Estate Recovery Bill. This gives the Department of Community Health the right to seek reimbursement for individuals on Medicaid after their death. This applies to elderly persons in long-term nursing homes or those who receive at-home care. This was the last state in the United States to pass this bill. The state was forced to comply with federal law or risk losing $5 billion, or 50 percent of the state's Medicaid budget that helps the elderly and the poor.

Under the new bill, nursing home residents who are current Medicaid recipients would be exempt from estate recovery efforts. Other exemptions also include homes occupied by spouses, minor children, or relatives with disabilities. Some people could seek a hardship waiver to be exempt from the program. A voluntary estate preservation program may be available where residents make payments to avoid estate recovery. The state expects to increase the number of estate recoveries over the next few years. This new law unfairly affects families of modest means. This is because nursing homes cost approximately $40,000 to $75,000 annually.

Michigan pharmacists lobbied to keep a new law concerning generic drugs for Medicaid from being passed. The law will base payment for generic drugs to pharmacies at a lower reimbursement formula based on the average manufacturer prices of drug and a 250 percent markup. This will force pharmacists to operate at a loss when filling generic prescriptions. It will either force them out of business or out of the Medicaid program. This problem particularly applies to independent pharmacies.

This year, Michigan approved a $9.7 billion budget. This would increase Medicaid spending in 2008 by $154 million. Besides federal aid, Medicaid spending would increase by $373 million in 2008. To prevent Medicaid funding cuts, doctors and hospitals agreed to pay an additional $60 million for an assurance program that draws on matching money from the federal government.

Michigan has several different Medicaid programs available for seniors and their families. One is called Supplemental Security Income, a cash benefit to low-income adults who are aged, disabled, or blind. It provides healthcare, vision, dental and mental health services. Another program is called Aged Blind and Disabled, available to individuals who are aged, blind, and disabled who meet the asset and income limits.

MiChoice is the Michigan waiver program that provides home-based community services to the aged and disabled. This allows individuals to remain home instead of having to settle for long-term nursing home care; the cost of care at home must be less than a nursing home. This program covers homemaker services, respite care, adult daycare, environmental, transportation, medical supplies and equipment, counseling, private duty nursing, and home-delivered meals.

The Medicare Saving plan is for the elderly or disabled with low income and limited assets. To qualify, you must have applied for Medicare Part A. Often, this extra money can be used for living expenses or prescription drugs. Some of the requirements are that you must have a monthly income less than $1,036 and assets less than $4,000 for a single individual. A married couple must have an income less than $1,390 and $6,000 for assets. This is a program for the elderly not in need of Medicaid.

Minnesota

The Department of Human Services in Minnesota and the Board of Aging has worked on a program to get health services for more elderly American Indians. They have done this through working with local tribal organizations. The need was found by surveying local Indian tribes. It was found that the home-based program provided by the Elderly Waiver and Alternative Care program was most needed in the state. Members of the White Earth and Leech Lake bands are taking advantage of the state's effort to help elderly Indians access Medicaid and home-based services. They are more likely to use the services if they can access them through tribal organizations. About 56,000 American Indians in Minnesota require services. This program is one of many designed to serve elderly populations in Minnesota.

The Elderly Waiver Program is a home- and community-based service for those 65 years and older who meet asset limitations and need medical assistance at the same level provided in a nursing home. Some of the services include visits by a skilled nurse, home health aide, homemaker, companion, home-delivered meals, and foster care. The Alternative Care Program covers trained caregivers, respite care and home care services.

The Consumer Support Grant is another program alternative to Medicaid home care services. This grant allows recipients to use some of the money for home services as a cash grant. They can use this money for a variety of home- and community-based services. It gives consumers more flexibility and freedom to choose services and deliveries than ever before. Parents, spouses, family members, neighbors, or friends can be paid to be caregivers. Grants may be distributed as cash vouchers or direct payment for services.

Mississippi

It is reported that Mississippi doctors saved $1.2 million per month in prescription costs due to handheld electronic prescribing devices. It reduces medication's costs and the quality of care because doctors have access to the patient's medical history, so they do not prescribe the wrong medications as often. Doctors can monitor patients to see if they are refilling their prescriptions on a regular basis. After several months of success with this program, they are seeking to expand it. Besides cutting down on prescription costs, it is saving on hospitalization caused by dangerous drug interactions.

Mississippi is one of the poorest states with Medicaid funding. They are addressing cuts in 2008 by discussing raising taxes on tobacco as a revenue source for the program. The state may be discussing Medicaid all year without a let up. The Medicaid program serves approximately 568,000 of Mississippi's poor and elderly, which some state recipients and social activists consider to be the fiber of society. It is the program that keeps the local hospital in business in Mississippi. If Medicaid were cut, healthcare advocates would almost certainly sue the state or fight the decision like they did in 2004. Some of the problems stem from funding used for Hurricane Katrina, which was one-time funding only.

The Division of Medicaid has approved the use of collected money called Civil Money Penalty funds in Mississippi to be awarded to nursing homes that provide high-quality care to residents. It will be given as an Enhancement Grant Award. It also gives facilities not in compliance a chance to use the money for programs that will help the nursing home make improvements.

The Enhancement Grant Awards provides money for improvements to nursing homes that have met standards for compliance for long-term care. It wants to give them money for the benefit of the residents to design programs that will make their life at the nursing home better. The grants range from $5,000 to $50,000. Educational grants are for nursing homes that have not been in compliance to design a program that will enhance the quality of life in the nursing home; grants range from $5,000 to $20,000. The money can be used for the protection of health or property of residents. It can also be used for relocations of residents to other facilities and corrections of standards not in compliance with federal law in the nursing homes.

Mississippi offers several alternative home-based programs for seniors under the Medicaid program. There are about five different programs under Home and Community-Based Services and Hospice Care. The Elderly and Disabled Waiver Program provides community-based services to individuals 21 years or older who need nursing home level care. A licensed social worker and registered nurse screen program applicants to determine eligibility. It covers adult daycare, home-delivered meals, and many other services.

The Independent Living Waiver program provides any individuals who suffer from crippling conditions that affect walking or the nerves. It provides personal care assistance for those who have rehabilitative potential and can direct their own care. Some elderly qualify if they meet the standards of the program. It is operated in conjunction with the Mississippi Department of Rehabilitation Services. This department also provides case management services.

Missouri

In 2007, Missouri Medicaid pushed through legislation that would increase payment to doctors and dentists in 2008. The 2008 state budget included about $25 million to increase Medicaid. Physician payments went from 44 to 55 percent of Medicare rates. A Medicaid reform bill requires Medicaid to create a plan to raise Medicaid rates to match Medicare rates by 2012.

Missouri Medicaid is now called MO Healthnet. It has instituted the Chronic Care Improvement Program, a program designed to help patients understand their illnesses. Patients will have 24-hour access to a health professional and information designed to help them; a signed release is required for Medicaid participants. It replaced Medicaid with a new focus on wellness, prevention, and coordinated care. It will provide health coverage to about 200,000 uninsured workers. Some of the improvements of MO Healthnet program are coverage of durable medical equipment on the basis of need and proof through an electronic information system. Individuals with chronic illnesses are being identified and encouraged to enroll in the program.

The new program will place emphasis on quality of care and patient responsibility. Credits will be given to beneficiaries who attend smoking-cessation programs, are losing weight, or seeking preventive care. Credits would pay for prescriptions not covered by Medicaid, health-club memberships, or even wellness coaches. The new program will reward doctors and hospitals that give high-quality care. All Medicaid participants must have a primary care physician. The program will also provide malpractice insurance to physicians.

During 2007, Missouri passed an estate recovery program. This legislation added a new rule that any resident enrolled in the Medicaid program at the time of death with an open estate could not close the case until they received a written release of the estate recovery claim from MO Healthnet.

To get a release from the claim, the following conditions must be met: the attorney representing the estate that the lien is on must fill out a report; the attorney must send the form to MO Healthnet for review. MO Healthnet will review each case and let the client know if the claim will be pursued or waived;. In some cases, a payment for an estate recovery fee will be required.

MO HealthNet for the Elderly, Blind and Disabled is for Missouri residents who are 65 years or older, or 18 years or older and legally blind. The monthly net income must be less than $724 per month or $970 for a couple. There are two nursing home programs. One is a supplemental nursing care MO Healthnet vendor payment. Supplemental Nursing Care provides monthly cash benefits to participants. An adult living in a nursing facility can receive up to $390 per day. Vendor payments do not provide direct cash benefits, but pay the nursing home directly the amount the resident is expected to pay. A person under this program uses all income for nursing home care.

Home and Community-Based Services provides home-based services to elderly persons who would otherwise end up in a nursing home. The program is for persons 63 years or older with a monthly income below the limit, which is now $1,088, and who need a nursing home level of care. It provides needed services like homemaking, cleaning, and transportation.

Montana

There are several programs in Montana under the Medicaid program. Individuals 65 years or older who are aged, blind, or disabled must cooperate with the Montana Third Party Liability by providing health information, completing a trauma questionnaire if needed for accidents, providing a social security number, and meeting the eligibility requirements. Another program called Categorically Needy Medicaid is for the blind, aged, or disabled 65 years or older. The income limit for individuals is $623 per month for single people and $934 for married couples. The Medicaid Needy Medicaid program takes it into consideration if income is above the limit, then the individual or couple will have a monthly deductible equal to the amount of the excess income. The deductible can be met by making a cash payment to the state of Montana. The Medicaid for Residents of Nursing Homes program helps residents who have income less than the monthly Medicaid payment rate for the facility they live in. They are allowed to keep about $50 per month for personal needs.

Nebraska

The Home and Community-Based Services program enables families with children or adults to stay together as a family. It assists elderly persons with disabilities to remain independent and participate in integrated community living and services. Some of the programs are as follows:

Adult Protective Services investigates reports of adult abuse, neglect, financial exploitation, and helps those victims. It assists the elderly who are unable to meet medical, nutritional, and hygienic needs. They must be 18 years or older and unable to take care of themselves due to physical or mental reasons. The service will set up medical care, mental health services, legal counseling, money management training, housing, and help with basics like food, clothing, and utilities. It arranges services for caregivers and family members, and provides respite care.

The Aged and Disabled Medicaid Waiver program supports people in their own home. They must be eligible for Medicaid and need nursing home level care. This program provides a service coordinator who helps you find the services you need to care for your needs at home. The coordinator helps you live as independently as possible. They assist you in locating housekeeping services, companions, and equipment to meet your physical and mental needs.

The Home Based and Community Services Waiver Program offers meals delivered to your home or apartment. The program is for those 60 years or older unable to prepare their own meals.

Chore Service is a service for the aged and adults with disabilities. It is to help them with tasks at home so they can live as independently as possible. They provide help with cleaning, shopping, preparing meals, and doing laundry. In addition, they assist with paying bills, simple repairs, and personal care. You can qualify if you are low-income, Medicaid eligible, and want to continue living at home.

Nutrition Services assesses your diet and helps you plan meals. Any elderly or adult who has special medical conditions like diabetes, obesity, high cholesterol, or renal dialysis may qualify. The Assistive Technology and Home Modifications program provides special medical equipment or changes to your home or vehicle to make it safer. It covers services that are vital to daily living needs including personal care, bathing, dressing, hygiene, and housekeeping, Many items are not covered, so check with the state program coordinator.

The Independent Skills Building Services program is for the aged or those with disabilities. They provide training with bathing, grooming, dressing, eating, mobility, toileting, and transferring. Some offer training for home management skills like housekeeping, cleaning, using transportation, managing money, shopping and preventing accidents. Adult Day Services is for adults with physical, emotional or mental limitations. Participants must be 18 years or older, and must need supervision and structured activities.

The Nebraska Long-Term Ombudsman Program was established through the Older American Act. It is an advocate for the right and well-being of nursing home and assisted living center residents. It provides several services, education, information, referral, consultation, individual advocacy, and systems advocacy.

The Advancing Excellence is a two-year campaign designed to promote excellence in caregiving in nursing homes and assisted living centers. It acknowledges the critical role the staff provides in providing care and monitors that care. Providers who participate must try to reduce use of physical restraints. They must reduce incidents of pressure ulcers, improve pain management for long-stay residents, improve payment for short-stay patients, access resident and family satisfaction, and increase staff retention.

Finally, Nebraska has a Telehealth Network, which uses technology to deliver health services and expertise to patients at a distance through the use of the Internet and Web-based e-health and video-based applications. For example, they place interactive monitors in the patient's home, often accompanied by measuring devices such as blood pressure, scale, and pulse. Patients' vitals and symptoms can be monitored around the clock. A telenetwork can be a hub connected to other sites. Patients can dial in through the network and have video conferences with doctors who are specialists.

Nevada

The Community Home Based Initiative Program is a program that provides non-residential services to older persons to market independence in their homes. One of the programs under this is Case Management, which provides assistance by licensed social workers to determine needs of clients and to monitor those needs. Another program called Attendant, provides assistance with personal care bathing, hair washing, toileting, and changing bandages. The Homemaker Assistance program provides services such as meal preparation, laundry, light housekeeping, and shopping. Other services include adult daycare, adult companions, chores, respite care, and nutrition services. Applicants must be 65 years or older and at risk in being placed in a nursing home. They must need assistance with bathing, eating, and dressing, among other needs.

The Homemaker Program is an essential community-based service that preserves the quality of the recipients' lives and reduces the need for out-of-home care. It is available for chronically ill, disabled, and aged persons who want to continue to live in their homes. Persons must be financially eligible for the Medicaid program to receive services. Through this program, the person receives help with a wide array of services.

The Long-Term Ombudsman program is designed to address issues and problems faced by residents in long-term care facilities. The program monitors quality of care, resident rights, medical care and treatment, nutrition services, deals with administrative issues, environmental careers, and financial issues.

The Waiver for Adults in Residential Care program came into effect July 1, 1993. Participants must be 65 years or older, disabled, and in need of an intermediate level of care. They must meet the strict eligibility requirements. They must be able to walk with a walker and get in and out of a wheelchair easily. Personal services provided are bathing, dressing, walking, feeding, toileting, and transportation.

Nevada has an electronic claims system for providers that speeds up the process of claims and direct payments to providers. It eliminates the need for envelopes, paper, and time that mail delivery takes. It works at making the system easy to manage.

New Hampshire

The Acquired Brain Disorder Services program is for adult and aged individuals who have suffered a traumatic brain injury or acquired a brain disorder. It offers a wide range of support services to those who qualify. It is a three-year grant program. Adults who qualify can receive day services assistance, community support, family support, and skill training. It is one of the programs available under the waiver program.

The Home Delivered Meals program offers meals on wheels to seniors in their homes. It is for anyone 65 years or older and disabled who needs help preparing meals. Homemaker Services are provided by the Social Service Block Grant, Home and Community-based Care Program and Chronically Ill Medicaid programs. The service provides homemakers to assist the elderly who need care to stay at home. The Transportation Services program is available for seniors and those who support volunteer activities including travel expenses for volunteers who are 60 years old and over, disabled, or chronically ill adults. Daycare services are available to some elderly one to five days a week.

The Congregate Meals program provides delicious meals in group settings to seniors and adults. Meals are provided in senior housing, church facilities, town halls, and senior centers. The program is geared to persons 60 years or older who need a meal in a community setting.

The National Family Caregiver Support program is a state and federal program for family caregivers in a variety of settings to assist them in providing care for individuals. This program helps those who care for the elderly with health or disability.

Some offer caregiver training and grants for respite care. There is also an Alzheimer's Disease and Related Disorder Caregiver program. Details are available through the state agency.

The Glen Cliff Home for the Elderly is a 106 bed nursing home facility that provides care for the mentally ill or developmentally disabled elderly adults. Nursing home care focuses on specialized psychiatric care for patients 60 years or older, and a return to the community. Individuals must meet the strict medical and financial requirements to qualify.

The New Hampshire Medicaid program hopes to move about 600 nursing home residents back into the community within two years. The Adult Family Care pilot program uses Medicaid dollars to pays individuals to move in and care for seniors in their own homes. It pays for non-medical services, but critics say that it does not have the resources to be successful.

New Jersey

The Global Options Nursing Facility Transition program is a cost-effective home and community service program that provides services to help nursing home residents find services so they can eventually return to the community. Some of the services available to eligible participants are assisted living, respite care, homemaker services, home-delivered meals, medical equipment, chores, transportation, and home-based support. It is provided to those in nursing home who are financed and approved by Medicaid. The person must have plans to return to their home and community.

The Jersey Assistance for Community Caregiving program is a state-funded program that provides respite care, homemaker services, home-delivered meals, chores, and other services. It provides these services to enable individuals at risk of nursing home placement to remain at home. The program pays $600 per month and up to $7,200 annually, after assessment of the individual meets the unique care plan and availability of services and funding. This is not Medicaid funded or under the Medicaid waiver program. Participants must be 60 years or older, reside in New Jersey, and meet other strict requirements.

The Adult Daycare program is a community-based option for medical supervised health services provided in an ambulatory care setting to persons who are non-residents of the facility, and who do not require 24-hour care. Medicaid does cover some services and individuals must meet certain guidelines.

The Office of Public Guardian makes legal, financial, and healthcare decisions for individuals ages 60 and older who have been determined by Superior Court to be incapable of taking care of themselves. It employs attorneys, care managers, accountants, and support staff to assist the elderly. They accept court-assigned clients because there is no other person willing, responsible, or appropriate to serve as guardian for the persons. The agency does not seek out cases. Sometimes, an elderly person needs someone from this office because family members or friends are unable to serve as guardians due to illness or other circumstances. Friends or family sometimes exploit, neglect, or abuse seniors who need care. This service offers help for those who need financial, social, and medical management in their lives.

The Office of Public Guardian employs care managers who make psychosocial assessments of the person's level of function now and in the future. They interview family members, social workers, psychiatrists, and caregivers to get the information needed. Assets and liabilities are examined in light of the needs that applicants require. If an applicant has limited funds but can remain at home, home care services are arranged for the individual. If funds are limited, an application will be made with Medicaid.

The Congregate Housing Service Program provides selected supportive services to low-income elderly persons or adults living in subsidized housing facilities. Some of the services include daily meals in a group setting, housekeeping, and personal assistance. It is a state program for the elderly who live in a community. They must provide one nutritionally balanced meal seven days a week in a family style setting. The costs of this program are far less than a nursing home.

New Mexico

Advocates for the elderly complain that a program to assist the elderly in nursing homes is not moving quickly enough. The program called Money Follows the Person allows some Medicaid funding for nursing home residents to choose to move back into the community. Medicaid will continue to be used, but in a home or community setting. One problem is a lack of funding to implement the program in the state. Another problem is not enough people to participate in the program to be caregivers in the community.

In New Mexico, proposed Medicaid cuts could create a $110 million shortfall for 2007 and 2008. The state Medicaid budget is $27.6 billion. These cuts would hurt hospitals that treat poor residents of the community and depend on this funding for payment. This is bad timing for cuts because the state tried to pass a bill expanding Medicaid funding for all adults within the poverty level. If the rules go into effect, hospitals could lose between $15 and $32 million a year.

Molina Healthcare of New Mexico gives incentive-based payments to physicians for providing good care to patients. This is a trend that many states have now. Molina encourages doctors to expand preventive services, improve clinical outcomes, and benefit patients. The patients are the ones who benefit from this type of program. Molina provides healthcare services for Medicaid and other government-sponsored programs.

In New Mexico, there is a Medical Assistance Division that has a Native American liaison working with 22 New Mexico Indian nations, tribes, and pueblos. They assist with matters related to Medicaid. The Native American Salud Managed Care Opt-In program went into effect on January 1, 2000. They receive Medicaid on a fee for service basis, unless they decide to opt in to the program, which means they sign up with the Salud Managed Care organization. A managed care organization coordinates the person's medical treatment.

New York

New York plans to promote a program for the purchase of long-term health insurance aimed at persons ages 40 to 65. It will helps finance long-term care in the state. The New York Partnership program combines long-term insurance with Medicaid Extended Coverage. It is insurance for anyone who may need long-term nursing home care because of a disability. It can be a wise part of financial planning at any age. The Partnership for Long-Term Care was created to help New Yorkers finance long-term care needs while avoiding financial hardship.

Some of the programs funded by Medicaid for the elderly in New York include:

The Personal Care Services program provides housekeeping, meal preparation, bathing, toileting, and grooming, For Medicaid eligible clients, these services are normally contracted through a home-health agency or provider.

The Consumer Directed Personal Assistance program provides services to the chronically ill or physically disabled who need help with daily living activities, or need skilled nursing. Services can include a personal care aide, home attendant, home-health aide, and nurse. Recipients have flexibility and freedom in choosing their caregivers for this program.

The Long-Term Healthcare program is a coordinated program for disabled individuals who need long-term care at home and are medically and financially eligible for the program. Participants can enter the program through the hospital or a healthcare provider like Medicaid. All Medicaid services are provided. Other services that may be available are case management with a registered nurse (RN), home-delivered or congregate meals, respiratory therapy, medical social services, nutrition, and respite care.

The Assisted Living program is for those eligible for a nursing home, but serves them in a less intense environment at a lower cost. This program provides an array of services like personal care, room, board, home health aides, nursing care, physical therapy, occupational therapy, adult daycare, and many other services. Participants must be financially and medically eligible for this program. They must not need continuous care or be bedridden.

North Carolina

Community Care of North Carolina saved the state more than $231 million during 2005 and 2006. It is the state's integrated health network that serves over 725,000 Medicaid applicants. It received the Harvard Innovation in Government Award. The program raised the level of healthcare and kept down expenses. The case management of the program seeks to keep patients healthy and help them avoid hospitalization and repeat visits to the doctor.

The False Claims Education Act requires any state provider receiving more than $5 million in Medicaid funding to educate employees and providers on federal and state law on fraud and false claims concerning Medicaid. They should be aware of the protection clause on whistle-blowers who report Medicaid fraud. Each provider will have to sign a Letter of Attestation to show they are in compliance with state and federal laws concerning fraud. Providers that have received a minimum of $5 million will be monitored and expected to show they are in compliance with the Deficit Reduction Act Clause.

Medicaid cuts could cost hospitals $330 million a year. The federal agency wanted to change the definition of the hospital for Medicaid funding, so 43 out of the 45 hospitals will no longer receive Medicaid funding. They are now seeking to only include the hospitals that have taxing authority.

North Dakota

The state received a grant of $8.9 million for Money Follows the Person. Participation in the program is voluntary. The grant will strengthen the rural area's community and home-based services. Those who participate must be on Medicaid and in a nursing home for at least six months. It will give the elderly more choices about how to live despite medical challenges.

Family Caregiver Support Services is funded under the Older Americans Act. It is for anyone caring for someone age 60 and older or seniors caring for children. Services provided include counseling and respite care. Services are provided free to those who qualify, and some people do pay for them.

Service Payments for the Elderly and Disabled program provides services for the elderly or disabled who are unable to perform tasks at home. The program enables them to live independently. It covers adult family foster care, case management, chore services, family home care, environmental modifications, homemakers, and respite care. The eligibility requirements are liquid assets less than $50,000, inability to pay for services, impaired in at least four basic living activities necessary to independence, and good mental health, including the ability to direct own care.

The Expanded Service Payment for the Elderly and Disabled program is a home-based service for those who would receive care in a long-term facility. It provides adult family foster care, case management, and chore services, among other services. Applicants should be Medicaid eligible or receive Social Security Income, and be impaired in at least three daily living activities.

The Medicaid Waiver Program for Home and Community-based Services is another program that provides services to the elderly who would require nursing home care. Some of the services covered are adult daycare, adult foster care, case management, chore services, environmental modifications, non-medical transportation, residential care, and respite care. Those eligible for Medicaid and 65 years or older will qualify. They must be capable of directing their own care and of living in their own home or apartment.

The Long-Term Care Ombudsman program is for patients in assisted living, basic care homes, hospital swing beds, and sub-acute settings. The program resolves and investigates problems and complaints reported in facilities concerning residents, and serves patients and families in long-term care facilities. The agency educates the public and families about long-term care.

Ohio

Ohio offers several programs for the aged or those with disabilities. The program is called Medicaid for the Aged, Blind and People with Disabilities. Participants must be 65 years or older, legally blind, or have a disability to qualify. It covers primary, acute, and long-term care. Ohio Home Care is a managed program of home care services for the elderly and those with disabilities. It has the Ohio Home Care Waiver Benefit Package for consumers who would qualify for care in a long-term nursing home. Under the Medicaid program, participants receive services that allow them to live at home including home-delivered meals, emergency response system, adult day health services, out of home respite, nutritional social work counseling, and care coordination.

In 2007, an Ohio Medicaid program expanded the assisted living program in the state. Now, Medicaid recipients have an alternative to nursing home care, as assisted living centers cost half the price of nursing home care. The state had to apply for a waiver to get funds to cover assisted living centers. However, fewer than 240 of the 33,000 assisted living residents are covered by Medicaid. Another interesting fact is that only 58 of 280 assisted living centers accept Medicaid payments. The assisted living center industry claims that the Ohio rate of $2,700 reimbursement is not sufficient to cover costs. The average cost of an assisted living center is $3,240.

Anthem Blue Cross Blue Shield will drop Ohio Medicaid by the end of March 2008 due to decreased reimbursement rates. The rates fell below organization's costs and they cannot provide quality care at those rates. This will leave about 87,011 state applicants without a managed care provider. The state plan that covers the aged, blind and disabled will not be affected.

Oklahoma

The state Healthcare Authority launched a program for healthcare management in 2008. It will benefit those with chronic illnesses and healthcare providers. Providers who cut costs and offer high-quality care will receive financial incentives. Providers will work with a practice facilitator. Patients with serious chronic conditions will work with nurse managers who will monitor them by phone or in-person. They will be linked between the doctor, patient, and community, ensuring they get all their needs met.

More than 130 nursing homes received bonuses through the Oklahoma Healthcare Authority for the Focus on Excellence program, which links nursing home pay rate to performance in ten separate categories. Some of these categories include patient and family satisfaction, compliance with regulations, quality of medical care, and staff retention. About 85 percent of the nursing home facilities participate in this program.

More than 5,800 members lost Medicaid benefits because they failed to provide proof of citizenship, according to the Oklahoma Healthcare Authority. The Deficit Reduction Act of 2005 changed the way states are required to verify U. S. citizenship to qualify for Medicaid. Federal laws now require documentation such as a birth certificate. Many of the participants received many notices and visits by social workers to get the needed documentation, without success.

Indian Health is a program available to American Indians through the Indian Health Services tribal clinics and hospitals and other healthcare facilities. They are normally identified by a CDIB certificate of degree of Indian blood, issued by the Bureau of Indian Affairs. Many American Indians prefer to receive their healthcare at American Indian health facilities.

Oregon

The Medicaid program will receive $1.75 million as part of the settlement with the drug company Merck & Company as part of the settlement in the case where the company did not pay rebates owed to the different states. Forty-nine states took part in the settlement. The company agreed to market the products under federal requirements that direct it to give Medicaid the best prices. The company manufactures the drugs Zocor, Vioxx, and Pepcid. This will put more money into the state Medicaid budget.

Pennsylvania

The state will not reimburse hospitals with Medicaid payments for serious injury to patients made by careless mistakes by doctors or staff. It will also not allow hospitals to bill the patients. The Department of Public Welfare will review cases such as operations performed on the wrong patient, medication errors, and bad blood transfusions. This addresses a growing concern over how taxpayer dollars are used in healthcare.

Pennsylvania has joined an educational program called Own Your Future, designed to educate the elderly on ways to finance long-term healthcare. It is an aggressive education and outreach effort by Centers for Medicaid and Medicare. The state plans to develop a unit to educate and inform the general public about ways to deal with long-term healthcare options.

A nursing home in Pennsylvania called the Holland-Glen Nursing home is facing serious charges for defrauding Medicaid and Medicare for shoddy treatment. The United States' Attorney's Office is the agency that filed the civil complaint. The facility was operating without a proper nursing license and provided care that was below standard. Several incidents occurred, including the staff failing to respond to the respiratory alarms, not administering medications properly, and treatment of beds sores.

The personal needs allowance of nursing home residents was raised from $40 to $45 per patient. This covers some of the items Medicaid does not reimburse or pay for. Most residents use the money to pay for personal hygiene products, phone service or cable television in rooms, bus fare for outings, clothing, shoes, haircuts, and greeting cards. This amount is not truly enough to cover some of the items needed for daily living.

Rhode Island

The governor of Rhode Island plans to divert money away from nursing homes towards home care services, assisted living centers, and families. The plans, if implemented, would save the state more than $30 million. The huge budget deficits led to this extreme proposal. The plan's goal is to give seniors more options and divert them away from long-term care by putting more money into other programs.

The Rhode Island Medical Assistance program is also called Medicaid. The Long-term Care program covers long-term nursing home care and at-home services. Individuals must be 65 and over with disabilities to qualify. The institutional services provide 24-hour care to elderly, which includes room and board, supervision, nursing services, transportation, recreational, and social services; Medicaid covers these services.

The Home Based Community Services programs are covered under the state waiver program, which is not part of Medicaid. Some of the services covered are assisted living center services, homemakers, home-health aides, case management, chores, and housekeeping. Elderly persons must be 65 years and older and meet financial and medical conditions to qualify.

South Carolina

South Carolina is looking to develop a new Medicaid

Managed Care Program for 2008. It would be part of the state's healthy connections choices. Privatization is a big part of this change, and the state hopes the HMOs (Health Maintenance Organizations) will cut state spending. About eight companies have signed on for the state Medicaid program. The program stresses care coordination and disease prevention. It seeks to cut costs by eliminating careless testing and prescribing the wrong medication due to lack of information and time.

Tennessee

TennCare is the program of managed healthcare that replaced Medicaid. It was implemented as a five-year demonstration program approved by the Healthcare Financing Administration. After 2002, it received another five-year period. There are essentially two programs: TennCare Medicaid, which is for persons eligible for Medicaid; and TennCare Standard, for those not eligible but not insured.

The Tennessee governor wants to shift more money away from nursing homes to home care services. He has proposed putting $12 million into alternative services for the elderly. This will help the 6,000 seniors stay at home or live in assisted living centers. Plans to shift between $200 million to $400 million from nursing home costs to alternative care are being considered. Self-directed care gives the elderly more control and options.

Virginia

Medicaid Waiver programs are different from the Medicaid funded programs in regards to the financial requirements.

They are based on the individual's income and assets only. Other sources of income such as individuals and parents are not included. An individual qualified for the waiver services is qualified for all services available to Medicaid recipients. If the person has regular insurance, Medicaid will be the second insurance billed for the services. The Medicaid waiver funds are government funds, and the availability is dependent on federal and state government budgeting and priorities. They are funded per slot, which is an opening of service available for one individual. Waiting lists are long and waiver funding is often limited.

Medicaid Managed Care is a program that helps those covered by Medicaid get the healthcare services they need. The organization is a group of doctors and other providers working together to give health services to its members. Often in managed care, the client can choose his or her own doctor, who will provide the needed services.

Wisconsin

The Department of Health and Family Services has an elderly benefit specialist to help anyone having trouble with government benefits. They can help the older person cut through the often-complex healthcare paperwork that they must deal with. Specialists receive ongoing training and are monitored by attorneys who specialize in elder law. Anyone 60 years or older or disabled, who needs help with organizing paperwork and understanding benefits can seek assistance. Specialists can help with Medicare Supplemental Insurance, Supplemental Security Income, medical assistance, and in many other areas.

The Community Options program allows the elderly to get the support they need to remain in their homes. It seeks to provide cost-effective alternatives to expensive nursing homes. Some of the services provided are home modifications, respite care, housekeeping, and personal care. There are no financial income limits, but the program will determine whether the clients or their health insurance will pay. The program will work with clients to find funding for the services they need.

Family Care is a long-term care program that Medicaid is part of. It is a flexible, long-term care program that strives to encourage people's independence. The program has a managed care component that is being expanded to offer elderly clients more services and support to meet their daily needs. Services and support include assistance with activities such as eating, bathing, or using the telephone.

Family Caregiving Information is available to help family and friends who are helping out the elderly. The network provides information about available services, gives caregivers assistance in gaining access to services, and provides individual counseling, support groups, and training to caregivers.

The Community Integration program helps the aged and those who have disabilities move from nursing homes back into the community. It is funded through the federal Medicaid program. It is an under the waiver program because the money can be used in the community to help participants. Some of the many services it covers are adult daycare, adaptive aids, case management, community residential setting, communications aids, counseling, daily living skills training, home modifications, and respite.

CHAPTER 10: Where to Contact Your State Agency

The Alzheimer's Family and Caregiver Support program was created by the Wisconsin legislature in 1985. It was created due to the stress and services needs of families caring for someone at home with dementia. To be eligible, someone must have a diagnosis of Alzheimer's disease and be financially qualified. The Wisconsin Bureau of Aging and Long-term Care Resources runs it. About $4,000 per person may be available, depending on county resources and budget. Some of the services include respite care, adult daycare, transportation, and support groups. For eligibility requirements, check with your state agency.

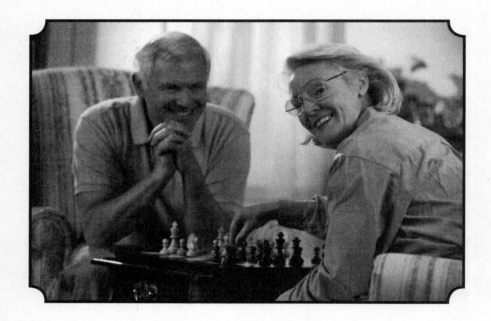

CHAPTER 11

How to Transfer Gifts

Old Half-a-Loaf Method

One of the most common methods to spend down your assets is called the half-a-loaf-method. A person gives away half of their countable assets. This results in a penalty period where you cannot qualify for Medicaid. You can use the other half for your living expenses or nursing home costs. Technically, you should run out of money by the end of the penalty period and qualify for Medicaid. As of February 2006, the half- a-loaf method will not work with Medicaid with a five-year look-back period ,and new rules state the half will be counted and make the person ineligible for benefits.

New Half-a-Loaf Methods

One method is when the Medicaid applicant gives away all his or her excess assets to someone as a gift. The person then applies for Medicaid and this starts the penalty period running. The friend who receives the gift returns half of the assets back. The person now has money to pay for private care while waiting to qualify for Medicaid. This may reduce the penalty period to half.

One problem with this method is that some states require the entire gift to be returned completely — 100 percent. These are called all-or-nothing states and this method will not help you if your state is one of these. It is recommended you consult a lawyer who has expertise in elder law and Medicaid for your state before using any specific tactics.

Another method is to lend excess funds to family members. In exchange for the loaned money, have the person sign a promissory note. They have to agree in writing to pay back the loaned money over a specific time period. Each payment should be equal and paid to the Medicaid applicant. They will use the money to care for their nursing home expenses. After thinking about this method and deciding on amount of payments, be sure that it is low enough to not interfere with the Medicaid applicant's income limits for qualification. It would not work if it disqualified the applicant from the benefits they are already receiving.

Exceptions to the Rule for Transferring Gifts

One of the exceptions is to transfer your house to your spouse; this is frequently never counted. The assets of both spouses are sometimes added together when one spouse must apply for Medicaid. If one partner has to apply for Medicaid, it is a good idea to transfer the assets or gift to the spouse who will remain living in the house.

A transfer of assets to a Medicaid applicant's child who is legally blind or disabled as determined by Social Security rules would not result in a penalty by Medicaid. The gift transferred should not interfere with the child's benefits. The best way is to transfer this gift into a trust.

A transfer of the home to the Medicaid applicant's child will not cause a penalty, providing the person was living in the house at least two years prior to the parent entering the nursing home. It must be the child's only residence during this time. The child will need to document that the parent needed to move into a nursing home but because of them, did not have to; a doctor will have to verify this. If the child lives less than two years, this exception does not work, especially if the person goes into a nursing home. Nor does it apply if they move out before the person goes to a nursing home.

A transfer of the home to a sibling of the Medicaid applicant will not cause a problem, as long as the sibling lives there for at least one year prior to the date the application is admitted to the nursing home. If the brother or sister owns some percentage of or interest in the home at the time, the balance of home is gifted to them.

In some cases, a hardship waiver will excuse gifts made of home or other money if the applicants can prove that not getting Medicaid benefits would be a hardship.

Trust for Sole Benefit of Spouse, Blind or Disabled Child, or Person Under Age 65

A sole benefit trust is a special type of third-party trust. It will not be counted as an available asset for Medicaid or Social Security benefits. It will not incur a transfer penalty as long as it complies with the exception rules.

The beneficiary must be the only one that benefits from the trust now and in the future. The money must be distributed and depleted in accordance with the person's life expectancy. Such a trust is only useful to limit the amount of money the community spouse has because of any trouble they might have in managing that money; perhaps they are poor money-managers, for example.

An irrevocable trust for the benefit of a blind or disabled child of a Medicaid applicant does not result in a penalty period. The child must be the only beneficiary, and payments must be made for the benefit of the child based on their life expectancy. Be cautious that an irrevocable trust does not cause the child to lose Medicaid benefits. It is good to have an attorney set up a trust for you. If the person dies, the rest of the trust does not have to be used to pay the state. Be aware that there is, at times, estate recovery for nursing home care for individuals under age 55.

Another transfer to a trust for persons under age 65 who are disabled will not result in a penalty period. It can be used for the disabled grandchild, sibling, or other family members. The person must be the sole beneficiary, and payments must be made to benefit the individual. It must be worded so that the person does not lose government benefits. There would be no estate recovery other than for nursing home care.

Transfers for Non-Medicaid Reasons

If, when you were healthy, you made a gift to your children or grandchildren, it may be excluded if you can prove it was not made to qualify for Medicaid purposes. In other words, you have to prove it was not made to qualify for Medicaid eligibility.

If you made a gift of a luxury car to your grandchild when he graduated from college in 2003, with the five-year look-back period, it would not even be counted. On the other hand, if you make a gift of a car and have sufficient income to cover your long-term healthcare costs in 2008 and then become ill, you should document this. In this case, the gift may be excluded as a countable asset.

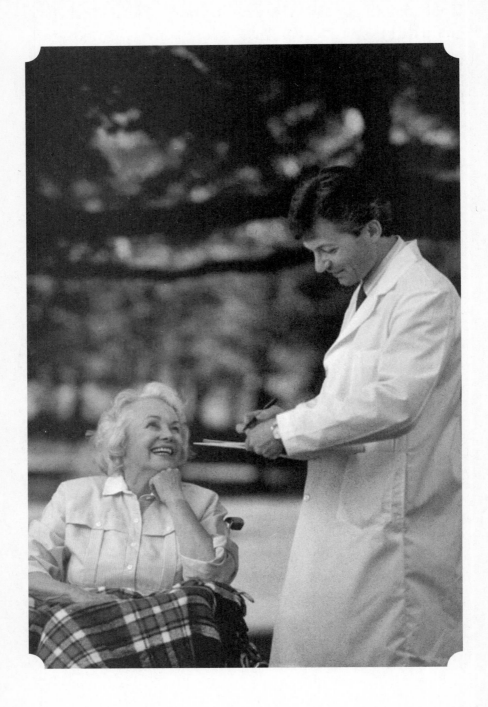

CHAPTER 12

Promissory Notes Explained

A promissory note is a loan or IOU. It is a loan of money that has to be paid back to the lender. When used for Medicaid planning, it must meet the following criteria to work correctly:

- It cannot have payment for a longer period than the life expectancy of the lender.

- All the payments must be equal in amount.

- The note will not be canceled upon the lender's death.

For the loan not to be called a gift, the person in the nursing home must have a promissory note that documents the loan. It should state the names of the borrower and the lender, the amount and length of the loan, terms of length of complete repayment, and interest charged, if any.

If the lender is a family member in a nursing home, the smaller the payment, the better. The payments will be applied to the nursing home cost, and you do not want the person to lose their Medicaid benefits. Do not make the loan longer than the life expectancy of the person in the nursing home. For example, for a female who is 75 years old, the loan can be for 12 years, not any longer; a female who is 85, can make a loan to be paid in seven years. The chart to use to calculate life expectancy is the Annuity Life Expectancy Table. The chart lists a person's age and the amount of time they are estimated to live. It is used to determine how many years an annuity should be purchased for. The life expectancy tables can be found at **www.annuityadvantage. com/lifeexpectancy.htm.**

Once you know the life expectancy, it is easy to find the monthly payment by dividing the number of months into the total amount. An example is a man who is 75 years old with a life expectancy of 9.24 years. He has $120,000 to invest in an annuity. Take the number of months in a year, which is 12, and multiply it by 9, giving you 108 months. Divide the $120,000 by 108 months and you get the approximate monthly payout that the annuity will provide for him on a monthly basis. The note must not be able to be canceled because even if the lender dies, the person who borrowed the money must pay it back.

You must name a beneficiary to whom payments will continue should the lender pass away. That way, it will not end up in probate court. If your state does not permit this, payments must be made to the estate of the lender. The unpaid balance may be subject to estate recovery by the state the Medicaid applicant lived in. The note must say it cannot be pledged, assigned, or canceled by the lender. Its only value is as a stream of income, not as an asset, so the state cannot collect it.

Interest Rate Charged on Notes

There is no requirement that any interest be charged on this loan. A universal rule to follow is that it is better not to charge any interest at all, which reduces the amount of payment back to the lender. The government says that if you charge little interest, there are tax consequences to this loan.

The interest on the loan is treated as a taxable gift every year from lender to borrower. No out-of-pocket federal gift taxes have to be paid, unless the amount comes to more than $1,000,000. It is best to consult an accountant to deal with the tax implications of the interest.

New Rules on Promissory Notes

In Georgia, a new ruling went into effect concerning Medicaid promissory notes. Promissory notes are popular among the elderly because of the easy and legal method they allow of protecting savings or leaving an inheritance while qualifying for Medicaid. Under this new rule, in order to be valid, promissory notes must be interest-bearing loans paid back in equal monthly payments. If it is considered valid, it will most likely be counted as an asset, and could make the holder ineligible for Medicaid. The new rule will affect about 500 families and save the state $1.6 million dollars.

New York State finds promissory notes a valuable planning technique. An example is a nursing home resident who has $100,000 above the Medicaid resource allowance. That allowance is currently $4,200. He makes a gift of half or $50,000. He enters into a promissory note with his son, and loans the child the remaining $50,000. The son pays the father a monthly sum that includes principal and interest. The calculations of the termination of the note will coincide with the Medicaid penalty period for lending the money.

The monthly amount to be paid is calculated. It is critical and must be properly calculated under the Medicaid rules and regulations. The terms of the note must meet Medicaid requirements under the Deficit Reduction Act.

The Deficit Reduction Act has put stricter rules on promissory notes and their use in Medicaid. It considered the use of a promissory note as a way to transfer assets to your children just to qualify for Medicaid as an abusive planning strategy. Now for the loan not to be treated as a transfer, it must meet three specific standards:

- The terms of the loan must not last any longer than the life of the lender.

- Equal payments must be made during the term of the loan.

- The debt must be paid when the lender dies.

Colorado considers promissory note countable assets for Medicaid. Under the new regulations, the person must get three estimates of the fair market value of the promissory note. Banks and savings and loans do not purchase these notes, so their appraisal is not considered acceptable or adequate. It should be advertised in a newspaper under business and investment opportunities. Three bids must be made to get a realistic value, and the highest bid is taken as market value.

Some notes have no market value in Colorado: notes with low interest rates; notes with incredibly long-term repayment schedules; or notes that are canceled at the death of the lender. These notes are often executed between family members to qualify for Medicaid.

In Massachusetts, promissory notes are still considered a good planning tool for qualifying for Medicaid. If the terms of the note comply with the three rules noted above, they are often excluded from being counted in many states. If your promissory note is considered countable and you meet the above criteria, you can ask for a fair hearing to determine if the decision made by Medicaid to count the note was fair and by the rules.

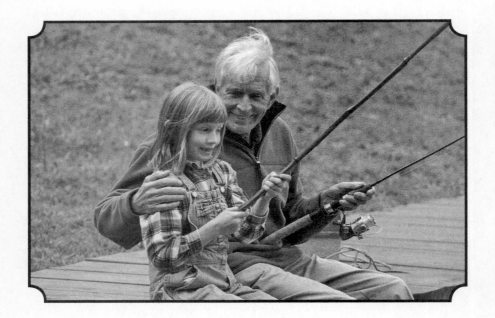

CHAPTER 13

Alternative Services to Nursing Homes

Home Care Programs

Many states are adopting home care programs in an effort to cut Medicaid spending. It is a new trend and many of the programs are slow to get started. There are different types of home-based Medicaid programs depending on what state you live in. Other government programs that do not come under Medicaid fund some state programs. We will discuss some of the new programs offered in the different states located in the United States.

The Adult Family Care program in New Hampshire was designed to move about 500 seniors from the nursing homes back into the community. The seniors will live with their families or others paid to participate in the program. This program was designed to cut Medicaid spending by paying individuals to take seniors into their homes and provide non-medical and personal care. There are two programs located in Manchester and Nashua. The providers for this program are relatives, friends, or strangers who are approved by the state to participate in the program.

The program began slowly because it takes time to approve licenses and do background checks on individuals who want to participate as caregivers in the program. The program is designed for seniors healthy enough to live with someone in the community. They do not need long-term nursing home care due to severe or chronic medical problems. The elderly participants have a registered nurse evaluate whether they can be moved into the community to live. The nursing home costs about $140 per day for a patient. This program pays $60 per day for food, rent, transportation, and the caregiver's time. Not many caregivers are participating in this program so far, but it is a start.

It is important to have alternatives for the elderly as to how they will live out their remaining years. For some elderly persons, one of these alternatives can be the best choice.

The Alabama Choices program began in 2007. This program gives seniors a monthly allowance for determining what services they need to live independently. Seniors use the money to hire someone to help with household tasks or for medical equipment or supplies. Financial counselors are available to help participants understand and manage the money for this program. Alabama is one of the first states to add this program. It gives seniors control over the home services they use.

Colorado provides some home care services under the HCBS-EBD (Home Community Based Services and Elderly, Blind and Disabled) programs for the elderly. The services provided under this program are homemaker services, non-medical transportation, personal care, respite care, electronic monitoring, and home modifications. This program is paid under the Medicaid program.

Connecticut has a program called the Connecticut Home Care Program for Elders. It is for elderly persons at risk of going into a nursing home. To qualify, you must be 65 years or older and meet the financial qualifications of the program. To apply, you must call and request the home care application form from the Connecticut Department of Social Services. If you are in the hospital or a nursing home, the staff can give you the forms there. The form will give you the details and provide asset guidelines to help you decide if you qualify for the program. You will have to have a health screening and have your eligibility determined by the department clinical staff.

If you qualify for the program, a case manager will determine what services you need to help you live independently. These services include:

- homemaker services

- visiting nurse services

- home-health aide

- delivered meals,

- someone to help with chores

- emergency response system

- medical services.

Minnesota has two different programs under the home- and community-based waiver program for the elderly. The first is called the Alternative Care program. It is a program for persons 65 years or older who need assistance, but not long-term medical care. It pays for trained caregivers, home-delivered meals, and household chores. The program prevents or delays an elderly person's admission into a nursing home. This program covers a variety of services for the elderly at home. The second is called the Elderly Waiver program for the elderly over 65 who need to be in a nursing home, but want to remain living at home. These clients need medical assistance to live comfortably at home. The program covers visits by a skilled nurse, home-health aides, companions, personal assistants, and also home-delivered meals and equipment modifications.

New Mexico has a new program called Money Follows the Person. This program enables the money to follow the elderly person from the nursing home back into the community. They must be evaluated to determine if they are able to make the transition. It is a new program that has had a slow start. The program gives the elderly person a choice of living in a nursing home or in the community with family or at a foster home.

In Ohio, many elderly patients prefer to live independently in their own home and near relatives and friends. Many entered nursing homes but the Passport Medicaid Waiver program has helped others stay at home. The benefit of the program is that it gives them a choice. Applicants are screened and provided with different long-term care options available in their community.

The second part is simple; once the elderly person is found eligible, a worker will put together a package of home care services that suits the individual person's needs. The person must be 60 years or older to participate. They must be fragile enough to require nursing home care, and able to stay safely at home with the permission of their physician. Some of the services provided are meals, food, transportation, and housekeeping.

More than 27 states received Money Follows the Person grants. This new program allows the states to transfer nursing home residents back into the community. Connecticut has received $24.2 million dollars to create a system to move nursing home residents back into the community. The program also uses Medicaid dollars for more flexibility, giving seniors more choices for living arrangements. Even 24-hour home care may be an option for some participants. This program funding covers assisted living centers, the family home, or an apartment.

Florida's Cash and Carry program allows clients to hire their own help and use the funds to buy equipment or supplies. Grace, an 82-year-old woman living alone, has many health problems and was never was satisfied with the help she received. Through the Cash and Carry program, she chooses the home care service that will help her and uses the remainder of the money to buy things she needs for herself. She is more satisfied with this program than any of the other Medicaid programs she has used before.

Assisted Living Centers

Many seniors and elderly persons live in assisted living centers. More than one-million elderly persons live in these centers who have mild memory disorders and chronic medical conditions that do not require constant medical care. Assisted living centers offer seniors a place to live independently, yet provide services like meals, housekeeping, transportation, social activities, emergency call systems, personal laundry services, and 24-hour on-site staff. Some are covered by Medicaid; many are not. Some assisted living centers offer limited medical assistance with medication supervision and other simple medical services.

Assisted living centers are also called continuing care retirement communities, personal care homes, and retirement homes for adults. Some of these communities have libraries, theatres, game rooms, laundry services, gardens, and transportation for shopping. Many centers covered by Medicaid have terminated their contracts, forcing residents to move to another facility after living there for several years. Many assisted living centers prefer private-pay clients as opposed to Medicaid clients.

Assisted living centers are a good alternative for those who need assistance but not 24-hour nursing home care. Families can live nearby and check or visit with the elderly person at many assisted living centers. Many families often live within 15 to 20 miles of the assisted living center. The cost ranges from $1,500 to $5,000 per month. Some expenses are covered by long-term health insurance policies and Medicaid. Many assisted living center do not use either.

Here are some guidelines to follow when checking out an assisted living center for a family member or friend. Ask some of the following questions:

- What is the building and surrounding area like?

- What type of meals do they serve the clients? Do the meals meet healthy dietary restrictions?

- How large is the facility and does your relative prefer small or large settings?

- What are the facility's visiting hours?

- Is the site clean and odor free?

- Are pets allowed to live with residents?

- What is the cost of the center, and do they have any financial assistance for residents?

Look carefully at the services and activities of the assisted living center before committing a family member. Do they encourage socialization and have facilities for this? Do the units have phones? Is it near a shopping center and a movie theater or other entertainment? Do they have religious services or a library? Does the kitchen have a refrigerator, stove, and dishwashing unit in it? Do they have adequate space to store the person's belongings?

What are the financial considerations you must consider? What is the cost and is a deposit required? What services are included in the cost, and what has to be paid for separately? Is the facility connected with a nursing home? Are utilities included in the cost of the monthly fee? What types of housing are available? Does the price of the assisted living center go up regularly?

Safety is another important issue for seniors. Check some of the following aspects when you visit the center:

- Does each room have an intercom?

- Are there exits for fires, fire extinguishers, and other safety devices? Is there proper lighting?

- Are there handrails, door alarms, and emergency buttons or cords for seniors?

- Are there readable signs on entrances and exits?

- Does it have air conditioning and heating? Is it a safe location with doors that are easy to lock?

- Is the facility in a good location? Is it near a hospital, stores, post office, and pharmacy?

Many assisted living centers accept patients who are too ill to truly live there. Before you decide on an assisted living center, make sure your parent or relative does not need long-term nursing care. One assisted living facility accepted an elderly man with dementia. One night, he climbed out the window when the temperature dropped to 26 or below. He was found dead from exposure the following day. He was not supervised properly at this assisted living center. Another patient with Alzheimer's disease was accepted into an assisted living center; he developed bedsores and signs of malnutrition after entering the facility for just a short period. These centers are not always equipped to take care of elderly patients with serious physical or mental illnesses. Be sure they have a proper medical staff before enrolling anyone in an assisted living facility.

There was another case where a man raped an elderly woman with Alzheimer's disease in an assisted living center. When you learn the facts about the incident, you will find that the man was a mentally ill patient with a criminal past who lived in the assisted living center. Both patients should not have been in the assisted living center because it was not set up to care for either of them properly. They both should have been supervised extremely carefully and constantly. The facility was investigated and found to be negligent to residents in many areas. That is why it is important to learn as much as you can about a facility before you commit anyone you know to stay there. There are many well-run assisted living centers, but some are not ideal.

It was found that in one facility, patients were often locked in there rooms. Residents were not fed properly and complained of not having enough food. It was found that personal care supplies often ran out and staff used paper towels sometimes instead of toilet paper. They advertised social activities that never took place. The state investigated the facility and found 63 violations, which tells you that this assisted living center was not regularly inspected. Cases like this have been found in Florida, California, Virginia, Ohio, Texas, and other states.

Seniors who need 24-hour long-term medical care should not be enrolled in an assisted living center. Anyone with dementia or Alzheimer's disease who needs constant supervision is not a good candidate for assisted living centers. Seniors with serious medical conditions for which they need medical and diet supervision, such as chronic heart disease, kidney problems, and diabetes, may not be safe in assisted living centers. It is important to know that a medical staff is on-hand to treat these diseases.

Most assisted living centers must meet certain federal and state guidelines. When you check into one for a family member or friend, find out if they are certified by the state. They should offer your client privacy, autonomy, and choices. There are a variety of laws that pertain to assisted living centers about services, delivery, and discrimination. The building must meet certain safety requirements, zoning laws, and landlord-tenant requirements to be in business.

The Informed Choice Legislation was passed in Oklahoma in June 2007. It states that residents can remain at an assisted living center as long as a physician says it meets the criteria of care the patient needs. It also states that family and patient must all agree that the needs can be met through the assisted living center and the community. This gives the elderly person a choice where to live and does not force them too early into a nursing home.

The state of Tennessee allows Medicaid assistance for their assisted living centers. This will give many elderly a choice of where to live. More than 40 states have adopted the waiver program, which allows some seniors to use Medicaid dollars for assisted living centers. The cost of an assisted living center is about half of a nursing home. Many state and federal officials view it as a more appropriate setting for the elderly.

In 2006, California decided to test assisted living centers as an alternative to nursing homes with residents who did not need strict medical long-term supervision. It allowed Med-Cal, which is Medicaid, to cover the costs of some residents in California assisted living centers. This would save the state money in Medicaid spending. Arkansas, one of the poorest and most rural states in the country, provides assisted living funding using Medicaid dollars for poor elderly clients who qualify. It has a large population of persons over 65. This state lured assisted living developers using tax credits, streamlined regulations, and flexible Medicaid reimbursement rates. This has lowered Medicaid spending about 10 percent in this state.

Last July, Ohio enacted a Medicaid assisted living program. It was expanded later to include those seniors already living in assisted living centers. The proposal was passed because nursing home operators often operate assisted living centers. Medicaid covers about 240 of the 33,000 assisted living centers, so this percentage is low. Only about 58 out of the 280 eligible facilities accept Medicaid residents. The rates are not what they should be, so few facilities want to participate in the Medicaid program.

Adult Daycare

If you are a caregiver or you have an elderly relative or friend who lives alone, adult daycare might benefit both of you. It is a planned program of social and health-related services offered during the day for seniors. The program provides meals and snacks as part of the program. Seniors who do not need 24-hour care are often good candidates for adult daycare centers. They must be mobile but can use walkers, canes, and wheelchairs. They must not be incontinent. Some adult daycare centers take patients in the early stages of Alzheimer's disease. Many programs do not provide the necessary medical assistance, so this should be considered before signing someone up for the program.

Some of the activities provided in the adult daycare centers are arts and crafts activities, musical entertainment, singalongs, birthday and holiday celebrations, book discussion groups, movies, and theatre productions. Some provide transportation to the center, blood pressure, and eye screening. This type of adult daycare has dreadfully limited medical assistance and supervision for patients. The average age is 72 years and older, and about two-thirds of the program participants are women. Also, one-quarter live alone, and three-quarters live with a spouse or other family member or friend. Family, clients, and charitable donations pay for the programs at these centers.

Follow these tips when deciding on whether the adult daycare center is right for your family member. Find out how many years the business has been there, and if they are licensed and certified by the state. This is important because they should be checked regularly for code violations. What are the hours, and do they provide transportations services? Evaluate their menu to make sure they offer healthy food choices, not just snack foods.

- Visit the adult daycare center and check to see how clean it is. Does it smell clean?

- Is the staff friendly and how do the other clients seem?

- What is the cost and what is expected of you if you are the caregiver?

- Do they have any volunteers that assist the staff?

- Is the furniture and facility safe for the elderly?

CHAPTER 13: Alternative Services to Nursing Homes

- Do they have grab bars and handicapped access for those less mobile?

- Are residents able to use wheelchairs easily in the facility?

- Is it roomy or cramped and overcrowded?

- What are the credentials of the staff?

The advantages of an adult daycare center include that it gives adult children with jobs a structured place to leave the elderly relative or friend. It helps ease the guilt of putting an elderly person in a nursing home if they do not have to be. It gives the caregiver a break from a 24-hour a day job that often has no relief. Many programs do not provide family members medical assistance with medications, physical therapy, or occupational therapy.

Sherrie's 96-year-old mother fell and had to have hip-replacement surgery. She had to move in with Sherrie and her husband Wayne. The constant care of her mother caused Sherrie fatigue and depression. Her mother agreed to try an adult daycare center near their home. She enjoyed the social activities and the yoga exercise program. It relieved Sherrie four days a week so she could work, clean the house, and be with her family and friends. The program gave her mother a life of her own. This is one of the advantages of an adult daycare program.

The purpose of an adult daycare program is that it provides a structure for the elderly. Even if they can handle living alone, it is healthy to spend time with other people in a structured environment. Even low-income elderly clients deserve to be able to have access to this type of program.

The Daily Living Center, an adult day center in Tennessee for low-income seniors, was afraid they might have to close their doors due to budget cuts. It was a place for the elderly clients to have a meal and socialize. Their clients decided to address the problem by holding a garage sale. The program was spared the budget cuts, but the effort the clients put into saving the center shows how purposeful some of these programs are. It was specifically designed for low-income seniors in Tennessee.

The schedule at the Daily Living Center is the following: Seniors arrive about 8:30 am for breakfast. When the weather is good, they go for a walk about 9:15 am or do an exercise video. They are provided with lunch and play games and have a rest period. During the day, seniors are always busy doing activities that are good for them physically and mentally. The program provides the necessary structure for these seniors.

Maryland has an Adult Daycare Program that is funded by Medicaid. Care is provided at medically approved facilities to those who qualify, including some seniors. Under this program, adult daycare offers many services including medical assistance. The funding for Medicaid and adult daycare centers varies from state to state. The Center for Medicaid and Medicare began a pilot program in 2007 that allows some money to go to adult daycare. Under the program, Medicare gets a 5 percent discount on what they would pay for patients' home health costs.

Tennessee Options for Community Living programs will pay for adult daycare and also the Medicaid waiver program. The demand for adult daycare is increasing by 5 to 15 percent yearly.

There are about 400,000 elderly clients served nationwide by this service. Medicaid pays for low-income elderly clients to go to the adult daycare program, although, many have too high an income to qualify for this program. Many states are passing legislation to get Medicaid funded daycare options for the elderly.

Budget cuts in Medicaid threaten some adult daycare programs for the elderly. In California, due to the expense, the governor has proposed a 10 percent rate cut for some programs, including those that treat Alzheimer's patients. He also wants to delay Medicaid checks to some adult daycare providers. Cuts in this program will have devastating effects to those whom it serves in the community.

There are different types of adult daycare centers; some just provide elderly clients with a place to go with structured activities, and are licensed by the state to operate. Others provide medical services needed for those with chronic long-term illnesses.

Adult Day Healthcare Options

Adult daycare health centers are for elderly people who need a place to go and treatment for chronic illnesses. They provide medical supervision in an adult daycare setting. They provide a program that keeps an elderly person from going into a nursing home. These centers frequently have several medical professionals on staff to oversee the care of clients who attend the facility. They often have a doctor, registered nurse, social worker, occupational therapist, and physical therapist. The medical components require that the facility have qualified medical personnel on staff, which is the difference between an adult daycare provider and adult day healthcare provider.

Adult healthcare centers must offer rehabilitation services with adequate room for physical and speech therapy. They must have adequate room for equipment with written treatment plans and assessment. They should have nursing services for monitoring medications and know how to use restraints properly. Nutrition services must meet health and sanitation regulations of the state. These centers must provide psychiatric or psychological services with plans for care. Recreational and social activities must be designed for individual participants. Transportation to and from the centers is often provided. There are some centers that provide special care for patients with Alzheimer's disease.

Alzheimer's Adult Health daycare centers should provide exercise and social activities for patients. There should be a registered nurse to supervise health and medications. There should be assistance with personal care. The facility should work with the family, physician, and staff to coordinate treatment. There should be transportation and good nutritional meals planned. Medicaid in some states often pays for qualified elderly patients for these centers. These centers should be licensed by the state you live in. If they are funded by any state or federal program, they are usually licensed to provide services.

When Helen, an 81-year-old woman with Alzheimer's disease who lived alone, realized she could no longer cope due to confusion and memory loss. She turned to her healthy, elderly, family friends for help. Mike and Loretta, a married couple, let her move in with them. They could not stay at home with her all the time, as they had other family and job responsibilities. A local day healthcare center provided Helen with the structure and care she needed during the day so she could live with her friends without being a burden. She spends the day doing simple exercises, participating in social activities, and eating nutritional meals. Mike and Loretta are free to work and spend time helping in the community.

These centers play a big role in relieving family members of the stress of taking care of someone with Alzheimer's disease. It also delays the process of having to put the person in a nursing home by giving the patient a place to go to get medical and social treatment. The patients are getting therapeutic and social care and giving the caregivers needed respite.

It is shown in a study by the state of California that many elderly patients with chronic illnesses use adult daycare health services. This includes the fragile elderly who suffered from strokes and falls. Elderly patients who have arthritis, heart disease, Down's syndrome, and brain injuries often use adult day health centers. Some communities will develop a particular daycare health center to help a specific medical population.

Here are some tips to consider when looking for a quality day healthcare center for an elderly family member or friend:

- Ask if the center is licensed and check to see that they have a qualified medical staff. The license should be posted or available for you to see.

- What are the hours of the program? Does the program accept clients with dementia, Alzheimer's disease, limited mobility, or incontinence?

- Do they have special services and medical staff for these medical problems? What is the cost of the program per day or week?

- Are there any discounts for lower-income clients and does Medicaid, Medicare, or private insurance cover the cost of the program?

- What services are part of the program?

Check on the kinds of activities the center offers for clients, Are there arts and crafts programs and exercise? Do they provide assistance with bathing and going to the bathroom? Do they have dietary services and regular meals? Do they have medical assessment, medications management, and adequate medical treatment? Do they have physical or occupational therapy? Are activities varied and geared to the client's interest? Do residents have input and help plan activities?

Are there protected enclosed areas for patients with dementia? What are the qualifications of staff members? Can caregivers or family members stay at the center with the client during the day? Is there a section for sick or ill clients to sleep or sit? How do they handle medical emergencies? How does staff handle difficult behavior?

Always check the physical environment of a facility. The physical environment should be clean and free of odor. What is the temperature in the rooms? Is it well lit and quiet with room to move around? Do noise levels stay moderate? Is smoking allowed? Does it have comfortable furniture with tables and chairs to sit in? Overall, are the building and grounds well cared for?

What is the staff like? How do they interact with other people? Does the food look and smell good, and do they have a varied menu? Does the center meet state and federal fire codes? Are there emergency exits, fire extinguishers, and built-in sprinkler systems in case of fire? Is the center wheel-chair accessible with ramps? How do they handle patients wandering off? Does the center offer transportation for appointments? Is there an extra cost for transportation available for non-medical appointments? Is transportation wheelchair accessible?

Adult daycare in the United States serves approximately 400,000 elderly persons. The average cost is about $61 dollar a day. It is about half the cost of daily nursing home care. It will become a viable alternative to nursing homes as the years go on.

Taking Care of Your Parents or Elderly Relatives in Your Home or Theirs

Recent changes in Medicaid make it harder to qualify by giving away money or assets to your child. Under the new rules, if you have a legal contract to help your parents out as a caregiver, this will not be counted as a gift. Many elder lawyers now draft caregiving contracts between children and the parents. Some are between other family members or friends.

The caregiving contract should specify the chores the elderly person wants you to perform. One woman set up a contract with her elderly aunt with the help of a lawyer. The contract specified that she would help with transportation and other household chores. All contracts should specify hours and how many times a month or week the service will be provided. Fees paid should be competitive with other home care services.

It helps with estate problems down the road to have a legal contract. The contract has to follow strict guidelines to pass Medicaid authorities. Consult an elder-law attorney to draw up a caregiving contract for you.

In 2006, a program called Caregiver Homes in Massachusetts provided up to $18,000 per year for caregivers to help elderly relatives live at home. It was covered under the Medicaid Enhanced Foster Care Program. It allowed family members and friends to give full-time caregiving to fragile elderly relatives or friends. It gave the elderly patients and their families an alternative to nursing home care. Participants must be members of MassHeath, also known as Medicaid, and need assistance with at least three daily living activities. Caregivers are supported by a team of professionals led by a registered nurse who is the case manager. They are given specialized training through the program and connections to other social service programs. Each caregiver is carefully screened and receives payment for their services to the family member.

There are many family members who live with an elderly relative and take care of them. Many are not paid, but may be qualified for this program and not realize it. For those who want to take care of their parents, this is a good option.

Susanne takes care of her 88-year-old father at his home. Her mother died a year before. Through an innovative program located in Massachusetts, she helps him bathe, dress, and take his medications. This program pays the individual caretaker or provides the participant with foster care. Individuals willing to take someone into their home must pass strict state requirements. The program targets low-income seniors in an effort to give them the option of living at home. There are similar programs in the state of Minnesota.

Caregiving can be frustrating and lonely, but for some, it is incredibly rewarding. Sometimes, it is a way to pay back a parent or relative who helped you become the person you are today. Sometimes, it is a deep commitment to family that makes one take on the challenge. Elder-care inspires some people to create or lobby for changes in the laws, which they would not have done this if they had not had a family member who needed help that they provided. Even if you cannot handle the caretaking because it is too physically or mentally draining, you can seek help. Never feel you have to do everything alone, and if you do some research, you will find that there are many wonderful programs and services.

If you are contributing financial support to your elderly parent, you may be able to get a tax break. First, if you are supporting your elderly parent, in order to get a tax break, you will have to put them on your income as a dependent. To get this tax break, they will have to meet the following conditions listed below:

- The person's 2007 income must be less than $3,400. Income from Social Security or disability does not count against the total.

- Any money from other sources of income such as pension benefits, interest and dividends from investments, or withdrawals from retirement savings plans cannot be claimed.

- You must provide more than half of your parent's cost-of-living expenses including housing, food, medical care, and transportation.

- Your parent does not have to live with you. IRS publication 501 has a worksheet for you on this topic. Pick it up and talk with your accountant or financial expert today. Please check with your accountant regarding these conditions.

There are different types of caregivers. An informal caregiver is commonly a spouse, child, or friend of the person. The person does not normally receive payment for services such as shopping, transportation, and cleaning.

Here are some tips on finding caregiving services for your elderly relative or friend:

Nonprofit organizations and churches often run soup kitchens and food pantries. They collect canned and dry food items so people can go to the soup kitchen to get food. Home-delivered meals and group meal sites are available to seniors 60 years or older. This is through a federally funded nutrition program. There is no fee for these programs, but donations are accepted.

The group meals sites, sometimes called congregate sites, are located throughout the community. They offer opportunities to meet new friends and interact with others. The centers sometimes offer nutritional screening and diet counseling. Home-delivered meals, known as Meals on Wheels, are available to the elderly who cannot make it to the meal site. Volunteers deliver a well-balanced lunch each weekday.

There are many small businesses that provide caregiving services to the elderly. They employ people part-time to help seniors with meal preparation, house cleaning, and other chores. This offers viable part-time employment to women and men, and also provides a needed service. The elderly will provide careers in nursing, social work, computers, and law in the next decade. Often, those working part-time with the elderly find it a rewarding job.

If you decide to have your mother or father or relative live with you, it is not easy. Caregiving regularly falls to women, but more men are now involved in the process. The caregiver's well-being can only be maintained by finding a balance between that role and other areas of your life; it is important to have time away from that role. Learn to pick and choose what you do and do not do. If your parents need transportation, perhaps you can find some alternative methods of transportation like buses for seniors or hiring someone to drive them. Their health insurance or Medicaid may cover it.

There are many organizations that support caregivers looking after elderly parents, relatives, or friends. These organizations provide up-to-date information including articles, and a listing of services that can help, such as respite care for the caregiver. Some nonprofit organizations even offer volunteers who help the elderly living at home alone. If you plan to be a caregiver, your local agency on aging may offer workshops and support for this role. Some even provide caregiving training workshops.

The local Agency on Aging in New York offers caregiving workshops. They offer caregivers a chance to meet others in similar situations. One of the workshops offered is Men Making

Meals, a cooking class for male caregivers where they learn to prepare simple nutritious meals. Other seminars are How to Balance a Checkbook and What's Under the Hood, a basic car maintenance course for women. So if you are taking on the caregiving role, your local office of the Agency on Aging can be a good source of information and support.

When your parent becomes ill and unable to take care of him- or herself, the first instinct is to have them move in with you. This is understandable, but not always the best move for your parent or yourself. You should consider some of the following factors before you take the plunge:

Do you and your parents get along well enough to be together full time? Is your home properly equipped, or is it small and cramped? Do you have the financial ability to help them out, or are you struggling yourself to make ends meet? What does your parent want? Often, they do not want to live with a child because of lifestyle differences that they are undoubtedly aware of.

Try the arrangement out on a trial basis for a limited amount of time — say one month. Be clear that this is a trial basis for the arrangement. You can even try the arrangement out for a week.

If you decide this is the right path for you, weigh the following considerations: Relationships are an important part of how families function. How will your siblings and relatives feel about you taking your mother or father into your home? Can you all sit down and discuss the subject rationally? Does he or she have friends who will visit him or her, or are you the only social contact? What are the limits of care that you can provide before you need outside help?

How will you adapt your home to your elderly parent? Do you have adequate space for them to stay, such as an extra room or addition? Do you have the assistive devices they may need like grab bars, raised toilet seats, and ramps? If you do not have these things, can you afford to add them to your home? Does your parent have a pet, and do you have room and the environment to take it on?

Financial considerations must be thought through. Stress over money can make caregiving more taxing.

What will be the financial arrangement? Will I expect rent from my parent or relative? How will my siblings feel and will they contribute to the parent's living expenses? Do I have resources to meet the bill with another person living in my home? Am I comfortable helping my parents bathe, or changing an adult diaper? Is there respite help available for me if I need it?

There are caregiver groups that meet to discuss the problems and joys of caregiving. These groups can be of help if you choose to be a caregiver. It is healthy to talk with other people who share similar problems. Often, you can share information and solutions to your difficulties. You will find that caregivers come from all walks of life and have a common bond helping out a family member. Members can share positive methods of coping with a difficult situation.

If you are considering joining a group, look at some of the following factors to decide if you want to join the caregiving group. Do you want a formal group that gives training seminars or a more informal group that meets to talk about issues? It is best to pick a group that meets your needs.

A group that has been in existence for a few years or even more is a good idea. A group that continues to look for new members is a positive sign that they are active and a good resource for caregivers. Who does the group focus on, the elderly or a group with a specific disease or age range? It is important to find a group that deals with similar issues that you do.

Finally, look for a group leader that has caregiving experience, so you will learn something new. If there are no groups where you live, do you have time to consider organizing one yourself? Some groups offer training in developing support groups so you can learn from experienced people.

The advantage of a support group is that it is a place to share feelings and experiences. You realize you are not alone and isolated, and that others share your experience. You can often get assistance and help, as others know something you may not. Some nonprofit organizations that help the elderly have support groups for caregivers.

Those caring for someone with dementia and Alzheimer's disease will find many support groups that address these issues. It is vital to find a group that respects your choice and offers help with doing the job you want. It is important to find a group that offers options for those facing caring for a family member. A group that knows about respite care and services for these patients is helpful.

Sometimes, a support group is the only support you will get for caregiving. Your family might not be supportive due to different reasons including not enough time or personal problems that interfere. The sharing and caring with the group can become your lifeline in coping with the courageous choice you made to care for your family member.

Call your local area agency on aging or senior center for referrals. Hospitals and community groups often can assist. Fraternal organizations such as the Elks, Moose, or Eagles often offer assistance. If your relative or friend is a long-time member, it can include home visits and sometimes transportation,. There is often transportation to and from senior centers. Veterans frequently can find a variety of services available through their local VA (Veteran's Administration) hospital.

Alternative Healthcare

Other forms of therapy that some doctors recommend is another option. Dr. Andrew Weil and Dr. Dean Ornish advocate natural rather than synthetic medicine. They offer programs regarding low-fat vegetarian diets, meditation, yoga, and group support. Other alternative healthcare options include massage therapy and deep-tissue bodywork, vitamins, and herbs. Holistic medicine treats the whole person, making lifestyle changes that help with overall wellness. Some insurance health plans cover some forms of alternative medicine.

Alternative medicine should not be used as substitute for regular healthcare. It can be used in addition to treatment to help with diet, attitude, and overall health.

Talk with your doctor before you use an alternative health plan. They often work with those not suffering from long-term chronic illnesses who need traditional treatment. It can often be used in addition to regular treatment for illnesses.

CHAPTER 14

How to Find a Good Elder Lawyer

What Is Elder Law?

Elder law is a growing practice and involves much more than just protecting your financial asset. It is a complex area of law that needs experts who understand the state and federal regulations that affect the elderly. This applies to Medicaid and other government programs that are designed to help the elderly with long-term care.

Elder law is growing field due to the baby boomers — a large population born between 1946 and 1964. This group needs lawyers for themselves and often for their parents. They represent the elderly person in many areas like abuse, neglect, insurance, long-term care, patient's rights, age discrimination, and asset protection.

Elder law deals with the preservation and transfer of assets when a spouse enters a nursing home to help prevent spousal impoverishment. Lawyers deal with Medicaid, Medicare, Social Security, and disability claims and appeals. Supplemental and long-term health insurance and disability planning are other important issues that elder lawyers can help with. Estate planning, long-term care placement, elder abuse and fraud, housing issues, and mental health are all areas that elder lawyers are involved in. Many specialize in certain areas.

When you look for an elder lawyer, look for one who specializes in the area for which you are seeking assistance; start with the National Elder Law Foundation. It is the only organization certified by American Bar Association (ABA) to certify lawyers in this special area. Anyone who is certified has gone through the trouble of studying and preparing to specialize in this area, as they have to pass an exam to be certified.

Also, look at the biographical information of the person. Do they have education and expertise in the area you are concerned with? Ask other people if they have heard of the attorney and what they think of her or him?

If you are going to meet with the lawyer, be prepared to pay a fee. Always ask what the fee for the first meeting will be. Be prepared to discuss some specific issues that are important to you or your family member. It is good to look for a lawyer with a few years' experience and in the local area where you live. You can ask for references, so you can talk to others about the lawyer and his or her skills. Take a copy of their brochure so you can study it.

What Is Certification and Is It Important?

The purpose of certification is to identify those individuals who have advanced knowledge, skills, and experience in the area of elder law. The lawyer must be certified to practice law in at least one state, must have practiced law five years preceding the application, and be member in good standing with the bar where he or she is licensed. Attorneys must have spent at least 16 hours a week practicing elder law for three years preceding their application. In addition, they must have handled at least 60 elder law cases or matters in that time period.

The attorney must have participated in educational seminars or courses in elder law for those three years. Attorneys must submit five references from people who are familiar with their competence and qualifications in elder law. Finally, the attorney must pass a full-day certification exam.

Tips for Preparing to Meet an Elder Lawyer

Prepare for your meeting or you may waste your time and the lawyer's. Not being prepared can cost you money because the lawyer charges by the hour, and will have to figure out how to serve you. It helps to have some notes or a list of what you are seeking when consulting the elder lawyer.

The lawyers will want to know who you are and why you are seeking help. Often, children contact a lawyer about helping their elderly parents. The lawyer will want to know the circumstances, and if any other siblings are involved. He or she will want to know why the parent is not the one contacting him or her. If you have power of attorney, you will need to bring the document with you to prove that you have authority to seek help on your parent's behalf.

Sometimes, a lawyer will send you a questionnaire in advance to gather information. Be sure to fill it out completely and send it there before your meeting, or bring it with you. Send copies to the lawyer's office or bring with you any copies of the documents requested in the forms you filled out.

Written documents are important to elder law. Some imperative documents might include copies of the power of attorney papers, wills, and trusts. If you applied for Medicaid, you may want to bring a copy of your paperwork to the meeting to go over. Spend some time thinking about what you might need for the meeting, and organize your paperwork.

Prepare a list of reasonable questions to ask the lawyer. Make sure you feel comfortable with the person before you commit to using them. Ask the lawyer what he or she needs to properly evaluate your case. Ask them to tell you how many similar cases they have handled. Can they talk to you about some of the problems you might face in your case? How long will it take to handle your case and what is an estimate of the cost? Does the lawyer handle the case or give the case to an associate to handle?

CHAPTER 15

Alzheimer's Disease and Medicaid

It is estimated that between 2010 and 2050, the number of people with Alzheimer's disease will increase from 5.5 million up to 14 million. The epidemic threatens to bankrupt Medicare and Medicaid. Medicaid spent an estimated $18.2 billion in 2000 for nursing home care of patients with Alzheimer's disease. It is estimated the cost will be $33 billion by 2010.

A study shows that about 14.4 percent of all Medicare patients have Alzheimer's disease. Nearly half of these patients qualify for Medicaid because of the high cost of the disease. At least half of all nursing home residents have dementia. This progressive disease normally requires some plan of long-term care for the person who has it, and the family that has to care for them.

Medicaid is the largest payer of long-term care for those with Alzheimer's disease. It is one of the few long-term care options available for this disease. Preventive care and hospital care are two required components of the program. The optional service is when the states offer more than the minimum required; often long-term care falls into this category. The optional groups include 80 to 90 percent of nursing home residents. When the economy is not doing well, these medical services are cut.

This can be devastating for patients with Alzheimer's disease who require long-term care and their families. The Alzheimer's Association calls on congress and the president to maintain Medicaid long-term care while expanding the home care options for patients like these. The group opposed the new plan to cut spending because it would affect this population and others like it who need assistance with long-term care.

The disease often takes years to progress. It causes a person to lose their ability to drive, work, and do normal activities that we take for granted. There is an increasing push for research to help slow the disease or find medicine to cure it. There have been federal hearings about the cost of long-term healthcare for victims of the disease. Research is not enough; we have to have long-term care options for families with this disease. It will not go away but become a bigger problem as years go by.

Financial Planning with Alzheimer's Disease

If you are employed, you should find out what coverage you have for long-term progressive diseases. If you do not have insurance, you should find out which ones have a high level of coverage for Alzheimer's disease. The local Alzheimer's Association can help you with this question. If you are over 65, you can qualify for Medicare and perhaps supplement it with another insurance through a private insurer; this insurance is often called Medigap. If your income is awfully low, you may qualify for Medicaid; this is considered a government safety net.

It pays to investigate disability insurance and how much it would cost. You may eventually be unable to work, so this would provide you and your family with some income for the time when you can no longer work. You can check with your employer or a private insurance company to find out the cost of disability insurance.

For long-term care under Medicare, you must have stayed at least three days in a hospital. You must be admitted to a nursing home within 30 days of discharge from the hospital. You must enter the nursing facility with the same condition with which you were hospitalized. You must need daily skilled nursing care. The facility must be Medicare certified. Your physician must agree and design a care plan for you in the facility.

Often, patients with this disease need home care. Medicare covers home care if patients are home bound. Care must be needed on a non-continuous basis. The care cannot exceed 35 hours a week or more than eight hours a day. If a person qualifies, they are entitled to a home health aide. Physical and speech therapy must be provided as needed.

If you have very low income, you may qualify for Medicaid. Some of the expenses covered include medications, care for hospital and doctors, medical supplies, health insurance premiums, and transportation for medical care. Medicaid coverage varies from state to state, and may cover home care services in some states. When you apply within your individual state, you will find out what medical services are covered.

Long-term care insurance may be an option if you have time to shop for a policy and plan. The policies have improved and can assist you with home care and long-term assisted living or nursing home costs.

Types of Long-term Care for Alzheimer's Patients

In Arizona, the Medicare Advantage Special Needs Plan designed a program for patients with Alzheimer's disease and chronic dementia. This health plan will offer residents special prescription drug coverage and care managers that specialize in memory disorders; the plan is managed through the health provider Evercare. The plan is designed to meet special needs of families dealing with Alzheimer's disease. This includes a care manager who addresses financial planning, support groups for caregivers, emergency respite care, medications, and other needed therapies. Members will meet with Alzheimer's specialists and have access to the latest drug treatments and methods available. This is a unique program developed for this disease.

Long-term care for Alzheimer's disease may mean getting help at home or moving your family member to an assisted living center or nursing home; there are more options available than ever before. If you decide to keep your family member living at home, some of the following services may be helpful:

Community organizations or residential faculties often offer respite care. Sometimes, families, friends, and neighbors can help. Adult day services programs are designed for Alzheimer's patients covered under Medicare or Medicaid and private insurance. They have qualified medical staff that provides programs and meals for patients. Always make sure they have qualified staff to handle this illness. Some programs may not be qualified but take patients when they should not. Home health services involve personal care with bathing, dressing, cooking, and other needed services.

Residential care options for Alzheimer's patients might include retirement housing for some patients in early stages who can live alone but not manage a house. It involves a small apartment, often with a kitchen or meal services. Sometimes, medical help is available from staff or a monitoring system. Often, social activities and other services are provided.

Assisted living centers are designed to provide some care, but patients must not need 24-hour nursing care. There are other centers designed for Alzheimer's disease, but make sure the proper medical staff is on-hand before you sign your family member up to live in an assisted living center. Specialized dementia care facilities may benefit those who need memory care assistance. They offer qualified medical personnel and special activities and programs for those with this illness. Nursing homes for those who need 24-hour care and skilled nursing are always available. Some facilities have special units for Alzheimer's disease with activities and programs designed for the individuals in it. For more information, contact your local Alzheimer's Association, which is an excellent source of information about programs and services in your local region.

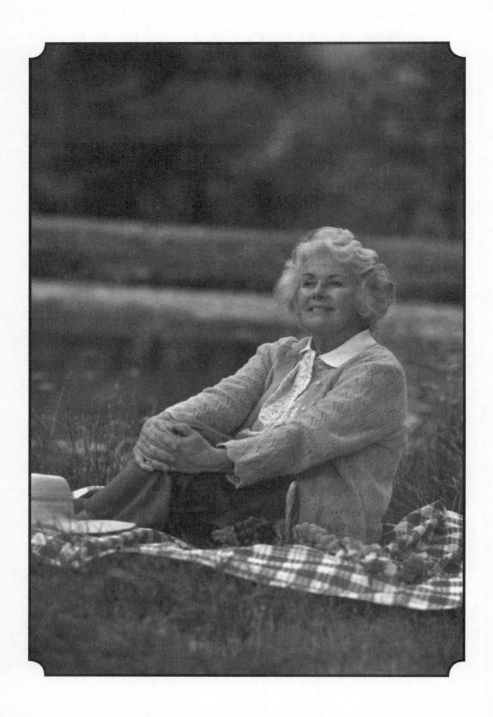

CASE STUDY: THE KARP LAW FIRM

2875 PG Boulevard

Suite 100

Palm Beach Gardens, FL 33410

www.karplaw.com

Phone: (561) 625-1100

Fax: (561) 625-0060

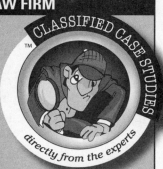

Joseph S. Karp, Certified Elder Law Attorney, Founder

The Karp Law Firm specializes in long-term planning for nursing home care, estate planning, wills, planning for special needs, disability planning, probate, and trust administration for the elderly. Mr. Karp is qualified in the area of elder law. The Florida Bar and a member of the National Elder Law Foundation, the only organization authorized by the American Bar Association, certify him as an elder law specialist. He was also a member and past president of American Association Trust, Estate and Elder Law Attorneys. His firm specializes in estate planning and asset protection for the elderly. They assist with Medicaid planning too.

Mr. Karp recommends planning in advance. The sooner the better now that the look-back period is five years for Medicaid. He says

CASE STUDY: THE KARP LAW FIRM

that Medicaid should really be a last resort. When talking about good trusts for the elderly he recommends the Irrevocable Income Only Trust. It gives the person control over their money or estate, provides protection from creditors, and allows for tax breaks. It reduces the risk of transferring assets directly to children. Transferable assets include homes, rental property, or liquid investments.

The solution to protecting assets is to transfer them to an irrevocable income-only trust. The parents can name someone other than themselves as trustee and direct them to give money gifts to their children to use for their own long-term heath care. The individuals can make themselves trustees and keep control over the money, giving themselves discretionary distributions from the trust. As trustees, they would retain control over what is transferred into the trust, giving them power and control of the assets. They have power to change the trustee if other than themselves and beneficiaries of the trust. They can receive income the trust generates but not the principal.

Mr. Karp says a benefit of the irrevocable income-only trust is that it avoids probate. It also allows a step-up basis or ability for the family to sell the trust tax-free after the owner's death. If you have the income, you can keep enough to cover the nursing home for five years and the principal goes to the kids when you pass away.

Mr. Karp strongly advises his elderly clients to purchase long-term health insurance as part of long-term care planning. Talk to someone about the different options. Don't wait until you are diagnosed with a serious medical disorder.

When purchasing a policy, look at the cost of care in your community your income and your assets. Make sure the policy has an inflation rider that covers cost-of-living increases. If you purchase a policy, keep it up especially as you grow older. Many elderly people will drop a policy at 79 or 80 when they are most likely to need it. Look for a Partnership Plan that combines

CASE STUDY: THE KARP LAW FIRM

long-term care insurance with Medicaid Extended Care. It allows you to protect some of your assets; however, in some cases, income is countable. When making any plans for long-term healthcare, Mr. Karp recommends consulting an experienced elder lawyer in your state.

CASE STUDY: DILLMAN AND ASSOCIATES

Attorneys At Law

1160 Silas Deane Highway,

Wethersfield, CT 06109

www.ctseniorlaw.com/

Phone: (860) 563-4070

Noreen A. Dillman

Certified Elder Lawyer Attorney

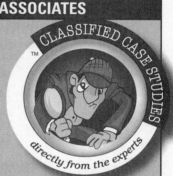

Dillman and Associates specializes in estate planning, asset protections, and Medicaid planning, taxation, and probate matters for the elderly. It is described as a boutique elder-law firm. Noreen A. Dillman is a certified elder lawyer with the National Elder Law Foundation. She is past president of the Central Connecticut Business & Estate Planning Council. The firm focuses on long-term financial planning strategies for the elderly and long-term healthcare planning. She advises anyone seeking to learn about trusts, wills, advanced directives, annuities, long-term health insurance, and estate planning and asset protection to consult a qualified elder lawyer.

Ms. Dillman describes annuities as an asset protection or Medicaid planning tool in Connecticut. She admitted it is hard to say whether annuities are a good way to protect assets with the recent federal law changes. It depends on the person's assets and the situation.

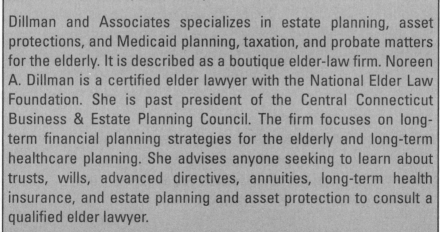

CASE STUDY: DILLMAN AND ASSOCIATES

On February 8, 2006, the Deficit Reduction Act changed the rules on annuities. Before that, there were none. Now annuities are considered an asset or income stream. Medicaid counts them.

An immediate annuity is a contract with an insurance company in which the person pays them a certain amount of money. In return, they send you a monthly check for life. In many states, it is considered an investment rather than an asset. If you have the annuity in the community spouse's name, it is supposed be excluded. It may or may not be counted as an asset by Medicaid in Connecticut. The law in this state is open to interpretation. Each case will be judged on an individual basis. The following conditions make an immediate annuity not countable in some states: First it is sound, irrevocable, and equal payments are made over a certain period of time. The state is named the beneficiary in the first or second position after the community spouse or disabled child. The annuity is purchased with qualified retirement funds. Benefits are paid out on the applicant's death.

A spousal annuity is not supposed to be a countable asset under the Deficit Reduction Act. This refers to an immediate annuity. Immediate annuities give a set amount of money. They are a combination of insurance product and investment. Connecticut treats annuities on a case-by-case basis, but warns using it —as a tool to shelter assets, it is a risky business.

Ms. Dillman advises people thinking about purchasing annuities to consult a qualified elder lawyer in their state. Dillman and Associates specializes in estate planning, health and personal care planning, asset protection, estate administration, probate, trustee and fiduciary services, long-term healthcare and housing issues, litigation, and administrative advocacy in Connecticut.

CASE STUDY: LAW OFFICE OF WILLIAM J. BRISK

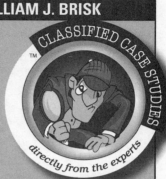

1340 Center Street Suite 205

Newton Centre, MA 02459

www.briskelderlaw.com

billbrisk@briskelderlaw.com

Phone: (617) 244-4373

Fax: (617) 630-1990

William J. Brisk, Certified Elder Law Attorney

The Office of William J. Brisk handles a variety of legal matters in elder law. They specialize in long-term care planning, estate planning, Medicaid eligibility, guardianship, and litigation. William Brisk is a certified elder lawyer and belongs to the National Academy of Elder Law Attorneys. He has a PhD from Johns Hopkins University in international and Latin American politics. He has taught elder law at Boston College School of Law. He has written three books on Massachusetts's elder law.

An increasing number of Medicaid appeals are necessary because applicants are being turned down more often. There are more denials of Medicaid funding these days than ever before. This is due to tougher qualification rules for Medicaid. When this happens, they appeal the decision by having a fair hearing with Medicaid officials. It is important to have an elder lawyer or legal representation at the hearing to get positive results. The five-year look-back period makes it harder for seniors to give a gift to their family and not have it counted for Medicaid qualification.

All states now have estate recovery for Medicaid expenditures. Your home is an exempt asset when you apply for Medicaid. If you qualify for Medicaid and have long-term care, after you die, if you still own the house, the state can recover the medical expenses. If your spouse still lives there or you have a disabled child under 18, the estate will be exempt.

CASE STUDY: LAW OFFICE OF WILLIAM J. BRISK

Long-term care insurance is a good idea for those who have assets to protect. Policies are frequently sold to people who have few resources and cannot afford the policy. You should not buy a policy if paying the premiums cuts into other basic living expenses.

Policies have improved immensely and are a good source of money for long-term care at home. He advises purchasing a policy if you have the money to do so comfortably.

He believes that most people do not need a trust. Some trusts are beneficial, like special needs trusts for the disabled, testamentary trusts, and some tax-related trusts. He believes many trusts are sold to those who do not need them. You must have enough assets to make them an effective planning tool.

The Law Office of William Brisk assists clients and families in facing the physical and mental challenges of aging. With two decades of experience, they develop sound plans, implement them, and when necessary, litigate aggressively to protect the rights of the elderly they represent.

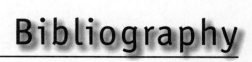

Bibliography

Books

How to Protect Your Family Assets from Devastating Nursing Home Costs: MEDICAID SECRETS by K. Gabriel Heiser, Attorney. Phylius Press, 2007.

Medicare for the Clueless: The Complete Guide to This Federal Program by Joan Harkins Conklin. Citadel Press, 2002.

The Complete Idiot's Guide to Social Security and Medicare, 2nd edition, by Lita Epstein, MBA. Alpha, 2006.

The Medicaid Planning Handbook: A Guide to Protecting Your Assets from Catastrophic Costs by Alexander J. Bove, Jr. Little Brown and Company, 1996.

Newspaper, Magazine Articles, Radio Stations and Websites

Senior Journal on Medicaid New Tech Media

http://seniorjournal.com/medicaid.htm

Piper Report Medicaid Medicare News 2008

www.piperreport.com/about.html

Medicaid Program in Fifty States

www.colorado2.com/medicaid/states.html

National Conferences of State Legislatures, the Forum for American Ideas, National Conference for State Legislatures.

National Elder Law Foundation Tucson, Arizona

www.nelf.org

New Hampshire Public Radio, State Pilot Program, Tests Alternatives to Nursing Homes by Diane Finch

Index

A

Agency 12, 16, 17, 25, 26, 29, 45, 87, 192, 194, 208, 209, 212, 213, 215, 218, 223, 259, 263

Alternative 12, 13, 20, 58, 62, 76, 120, 140, 143, 171, 172, 181, 192, 198, 199, 216, 220, 242, 246, 255, 256, 259, 263

Alzheimer 77, 177, 181, 185, 190, 208, 223-245, 247, 251-253, 262, 269, 270, 272, 273

Annuity 79-89, 123, 232, 278

Application 17, 26, 53, 56, 76, 134, 210, 227, 239, 267

Assets 11-13, 16, 25-27, 29-31, 33, 34, 36-41, 43, 44, 46-48, 50-52, 54-67, 69-72, 74, 80, 82, 83, 85, 86, 88, 92, 93, 95-97, 100, 101, 103, 104, 106, 107, 111, 115, 117, 118, 122-126, 130, 133, 139, 140, 142, 179, 196, 197, 214, 221, 225, 226, 234, 255, 265, 276, 277, 278, 280

Assistance 15, 150, 153, 158, 159, 161, 164, 169, 175, 205, 209, 211, 212, 219

B

Behavior 177, 254

Beneficiary 55, 61, 63, 71, 79-81, 84, 88, 89, 106, 109, 110, 112, 227, 228, 232, 278

Bills 18, 19, 25, 26, 28, 69, 112, 117, 120, 124, 142, 168, 204

Bypass 24, 108

C

Caretaker 256

Certification 74, 266

Cost 11, 12, 16, 19, 20, 25, 27, 29, 41, 46, 47, 53, 69, 72, 75, 80, 85, 92, 94, 98-111, 116, 118-120, 122, 136, 142, 166, 179, 182, 184, 188, 190, 193-196, 208, 212, 213, 216, 222, 231, 242, 243, 246, 248, 254, 255, 258, 267-271, 276

Court 38, 52, 61, 65, 68, 77,

105, 106, 124, 136-139, 209, 232

Creditor 45, 52, 59

Cuts 40, 98, 167, 186, 189-191, 196, 198, 210, 211, 213, 250, 251, 280

D

Deductible 100, 121, 122, 182, 202

Deed 48-50, 65, 95, 107-111, 123, 133, 135-139

Diabetes 23, 24, 181, 185, 204, 245

Disabled 13, 15, 16, 21, 26, 27, 35, 43-45, 51-53, 57, 59, 61-63, 65, 66, 88, 89, 92, 100, 118, 120, 137, 166-172, 176-178, 182-185, 192, 196, 202, 206-208, 212, 214, 216, 221, 226, 228, 278-280

Doctor 18, 23, 24, 28, 72, 74, 75, 77, 115, 116, 142, 144, 146, 169, 178, 180, 186, 213, 216, 221, 227, 251, 263

Drugs 18, 28, 115, 116, 166, 167, 170, 173, 180-183, 194, 195, 197, 217

E

Elderly 12, 13, 15, 16, 19-23, 30, 56, 59, 60, 62, 66, 78, 87, 101, 120, 124, 125, 127, 129, 141-145, 166, 167, 169-171, 173-177, 179-185, 187-193, 195-198, 200, 202-204, 207-210, 212, 214, 215, 218-222, 233, 238-242, 244-253, 255-259, 261, 262, 265, 267, 275-277, 280

Equipment 20, 28, 128, 144, 166, 173, 187, 196, 200, 203, 204, 208, 238, 240, 241, 252

Estate 39, 43-47, 49-54, 56, 57, 58, 61, 63, 64, 66, 68-70, 73, 74, 78, 86, 89, 94, 95, 97, 101, 107-110, 112, 124, 125, 130, 134-136, 138-140, 142, 146, 179, 195, 201, 228, 232, 256, 275-280

F

Family 11, 12, 18-21, 24, 25, 30, 36-38, 43-47, 50, 56, 57, 60, 62, 63, 65, 69, 72, 73, 75, 77, 84, 86, 88, 91, 92, 94-96, 98, 99, 101, 102, 105, 107, 109, 112, 113, 116, 118-120, 123-125, 127-131, 133, 134, 140-143, 146, 176, 182, 185, 198, 203, 205, 207-210, 214, 217, 222, 226, 228, 231, 235, 240-243, 246, 248, 249, 252-257, 261-263, 266, 269, 271-273, 276, 279

G

Gift 40, 41, 49, 50, 55, 56, 58-

60, 64, 67, 68, 70, 71, 72, 87, 91-94, 96, 97, 100-102, 109, 110, 129, 130, 134-136, 139-141, 225, 226, 228, 229, 231, 233, 255, 279

Government 15, 18, 25, 63, 66, 71, 97, 117, 168, 186, 188-191, 196, 211, 221, 228, 233, 237, 265, 270

Guardian 61, 65, 66, 104, 209

H

HCBS 13, 18-22, 45, 173, 183, 184, 238

Health 11, 12, 15, 18-24, 28, 43, 63, 73, 76, 82, 84, 85, 95, 98, 99, 101, 115, 119, 120, 122, 127, 139, 146, 147, 159, 163, 166-169, 172, 173, 175, 178, 179, 182, 183, 189, 194-197, 199-203, 205, 208, 209, 211-215, 217, 219, 221, 222, 239-242, 247, 250-253, 259, 263, 265, 266, 271-273, 276, 277, 278

Healthcare 11, 43, 47, 72-78, 97, 98, 103, 115, 121, 166, 167, 168, 170, 173, 175, 176, 178, 181, 182, 184-186, 189, 191-194, 196, 198, 209, 211-213, 216-218, 220, 221, 229, 252, 253, 263, 270, 277, 278

Heart disease 24, 245, 253

Home-based 12, 142, 190, 193, 196, 197, 199, 202, 208, 214, 237

Hospice 199

Hospital 16, 18, 53, 75, 78, 100, 169, 171, 173, 176, 180, 187, 198, 212, 213, 215, 239, 244, 263, 269, 271

I

Income 11, 15-18, 25-31, 34, 40, 47, 55, 57-60, 63, 64, 66, 69, 70, 72, 80, 82-89, 91, 96, 97, 101, 115, 117-119, 123, 124, 126, 130, 131, 134, 146, 167, 169, 172-174, 177-182, 187, 190, 194, 196, 197, 201, 202, 204, 210, 221, 222, 226, 229, 232, 250, 251, 254, 257, 270, 271, 276-278

Insurance 11, 15, 16, 26, 28, 30, 31, 33, 34, 37, 38, 43, 51, 53, 56, 60, 66-68, 79, 80, 82-85, 93, 97, 98, 101, 115, 119-122, 135, 169, 177, 182, 183, 194, 195, 201, 211, 221, 222, 242, 254, 259, 263, 265, 270-273, 276-278, 280

Issues 12, 13, 63, 109, 112, 138, 145, 178, 206, 261, 262, 265, 266, 278

L

Lawyer 11-13, 27, 49, 74, 77, 82, 83, 87, 88, 95, 104,

112, 139, 142, 226, 255, 266-268, 277-279

Liens 45, 50

Living will 73-76, 78

Loans 111, 233, 234

M

Married 28, 35, 37, 39, 46, 57, 61, 69, 82, 83, 92, 96, 110, 111, 134, 135, 197, 202, 252

Meals 19-21, 24, 125, 128, 145, 170, 175, 183, 196, 197, 200, 203, 204, 207-210, 212, 215, 239-243, 247, 252-254, 258, 260, 273

Medical coverage 15, 16, 45

MMMNA 29, 30, 89

Money 12, 16, 19, 20, 25-31, 33, 36-40, 45, 46, 51, 54, 56, 58-63, 65-67, 70, 72, 78, 82-86, 88, 89, 91-98, 102, 104, 106, 111, 112, 116-119, 123, 124, 126, 128, 129, 134, 137, 144-146, 166, 167, 169-171, 173, 174, 177, 178, 183-188, 190, 191, 196-199, 203, 204, 218-220, 222, 225-228, 231, 232, 234, 238, 240, 241, 246, 250, 255, 257, 261, 267, 276, 278, 280

N

Nurse 18, 24, 27, 116, 178, 197, 199, 212, 216, 238,

239, 240, 251, 252, 256

Nutrition 204, 252

P

Penalty 92, 199

Physician 200

Poor 15, 173, 177, 194, 195, 198, 210, 228, 247

Prepare 12, 13, 72, 73, 74, 103, 112, 128, 203, 260

Prescription 18, 28, 53, 116, 166, 167, 170, 173, 180-182, 197, 198, 272

Program 11, 13, 15-18, 20-25, 51, 52, 53, 55, 117, 127, 128, 142, 166, 169-188, 190-223, 237-241, 246-258, 269, 272

Property 27, 29, 36, 38-40, 45-53, 56-58, 63, 65, 69, 78, 92, 94, 101-104, 106-112, 118, 124, 127, 133-140, 146, 169, 199, 276

Q

Qualification 28, 226, 279

R

Recipient 12, 38, 44-46, 51, 52, 88, 102, 133, 179, 190

Record 26, 49, 52

Rehab 20

Relief 22, 249

Resources 31, 55, 60, 61, 167-169, 173, 208, 223, 261, 280

Rules 11, 12, 28, 29, 34, 40, 44, 50, 51, 54, 60, 71, 82,

87, 92, 93, 96, 98, 100,
111, 141, 142, 144, 145,
189, 191, 211, 225, 226,
227, 234, 235, 255, 278,
279

S

Senior 12, 20, 127, 129, 144,
183, 207, 263
Single 27, 28, 35, 37, 57, 82,
83, 87, 88, 92, 122, 169,
194, 197, 202
Social Security 15, 17, 21, 27-
30, 44, 45, 50, 52, 57, 61,
126, 174, 177, 214, 226,
227, 257, 265
Spouse 29-31, 35-40, 43-46,
48, 50-55, 57-59, 61, 62,
67, 69, 81, 82, 84, 88, 89,
91, 92, 95, 96, 100, 103,
106, 107, 110, 112, 124,
126, 130, 136, 143, 169,
179, 226, 228, 248, 258,
265, 278, 279
States 11, 12, 15-23, 25, 27,
37-40, 43-47, 51, 52, 55,
61, 65, 66, 69, 70, 71, 73,
74, 80, 82, 87, 89, 91, 93,
98, 103-105, 107-109,
125, 129, 143, 166-168,
186, 190, 192, 198, 211,
217, 226, 235, 237, 238,
241, 245-247, 251, 252,
269, 271, 278, 279
Survivor 46, 49, 84

T

Taxes 27, 30, 58, 60, 63, 65,
68, 69, 82, 83, 86, 96, 97,
101, 102, 112, 130, 135,
136, 138-140, 143, 146,
198, 233
Tired 24
Transfer 19, 24, 38, 40, 47,
49, 54, 55, 58, 60, 64, 65,
68, 71, 82, 86, 91, 92, 94,
96, 101, 102, 107, 108,
123, 133-141, 226-228,
234, 241, 265, 276
Trustee 56-60, 63, 65-69, 72,
112, 113, 276, 278
Trusts 26, 56, 58, 63-66, 69,
71, 72, 95, 97, 108, 268,
276, 277, 280

V

Value 33-38, 46, 47, 50, 56,
67, 69, 80, 82, 85-87,
91-94, 102, 108, 110, 118,
122, 129, 130, 134, 135,
139, 140, 146, 182, 232,
234, 235

W

Waiver 93, 152, 167, 171,
172, 175, 182, 183, 197,
199, 200, 203, 206, 215,
221, 240
Will 11, 12, 18, 19, 21, 25,
27-31, 34-36, 40, 43-48,
50, 52, 54, 55, 57, 58-63,
65-68, 70-89, 91-101,
103-109, 111, 117-120,
122-126, 129, 133-138,
140-146, 167, 168, 170,
173-175, 177-179, 183-

193, 195, 196, 199, 200-
203, 210, 211, 213-218,
220-222, 225-228, 231-
234, 237-241, 245, 246,
250, 251, 253, 255, 257,
259-262, 266-272, 276,
278, 280